WORKBOOK

Guide to Good Food

INSTRUCTOR'S ANNOTATED WORKBOOK

13th Edition

Deborah L. Bence
Family and Consumer Sciences Author
Granville, Ohio

Guide to Good Food Text
by Velda L. Largen and Deborah L. Bence

Publisher
The Goodheart-Willcox Company, Inc.
Tinley Park, Illinois
www.g-w.com

INTRODUCTION

This Workbook is designed for use with the text **Guide to Good Food**. It will help you understand and remember the facts and concepts about food and nutrition presented in the text. It will also help you apply this learning in your daily life.

The activities in this workbook are divided into chapters that correspond to the chapters in the text. By reading the text first, you will have the information you need to complete the activities. Try to complete the activities without referring to the text. If necessary, you can look at the book again later to complete any questions you could not answer. At that time, you can also compare the answers you have to the information in the book.

You will find a number of activities in this workbook. Many of the activities, such as crossword puzzles, true and false questions, and fill-in-the-blank sentences, have *right* answers. These activities can be used as review guides when you study for tests and quizzes. Other activities, such as evaluations and comparisons, will ask for opinions and ideas that cannot be judged as *right* or *wrong*. These activities are designed to stimulate your thinking and help you apply information presented in the text.

The activities in this workbook have been designed to increase your interest and understanding of the text material. The more thought you put into the activities, the more knowledge you will gain from them.

CONTENTS

Part 2   The Management of Food

Part 3   The Preparation of Food

Part 4   Food and Careers

Part 5   Foods of the World

CHAPTER 1
Food Affects Life

Making Food Decisions

Activity A   Name ____

Chapter 1   Date _______________________   Period_______________________

Think of a specific issue about buying, preparing, or ordering food. Complete the following exercise to help work through the steps of the decision-making process. Write your answers in the space provided.

1. **Identify the problem or decision.** (Answers will vary.) _______________________

   ____

2. **Consider your alternatives.** List three options from which you might choose.

   A. (Answers will vary.) ____

   B. (Answers will vary.) ____

   C. (Answers will vary.) ____

3. **Think about how your alternatives relate to your goals.** Identify one or more goals you have related to this issue.

   (Answers will vary.) ____

   ____

   ____

4. **Determine which alternatives are acceptable.** For each of the alternatives you listed in Step 2, place a check in front of the corresponding letter below if you feel the alternative is suitable when measured against your goal(s). If an alternative is not acceptable, explain why in the space following the corresponding letter below.

   _______ A. (Answers will vary.) ____

   _______ B. (Answers will vary.) ____

   _______ C. (Answers will vary.) ____

5. **Choose one alternative.** Place a check in front of the letter that corresponds to the alternative you will choose. Then explain why you chose this alternative.

   _______ A   _______ B   _______ C

   (Answers will vary.) ____

   ____

6. **Evaluate your decision.** How did this decision help you meet your goals? How might this decision help you make decisions in the future?

   (Answers will vary.) ____

   ____

Advertising Analysis

Activity B   **Name** ____

Chapter 1   **Date** _______________________   **Period** ____________________

Clip an advertisement for a food product from a newspaper or magazine and attach it to this page. Then answer the following questions about the advertisement in the space provided.

1. What about this advertisement first caught your eye? _(Answers will vary.)_________

____

2. What is the brand of the advertised product? _(Answers will vary.)_____________

3. What is the name of the advertised product?_(Answers will vary.)_______________

4. Is this a new food product or one that has been available for some time? _(Answers will vary.)______

5. What impressions do you get from the photos and colors used on the product packaging?

_(Answers will vary.)____

____

6. Describe the technique(s) this advertisement uses to encourage people to buy this product.

_(Answers will vary.)____

____

____

7. What, if any, advertising icons are associated with this product? _(Answers will vary.)______

8. What useful information does this advertisement give you about the product? _______________

_(Answers will vary.)____

____

____

9. Would you likely talk to others about this advertisement? Explain why or why not. _______________

_(Answers will vary.)____

____

10. After seeing this advertisement, would you be interested in using this product? Explain why or why not.

_(Answers will vary.)____

____

11. What, if any, other products are you aware of that are made by the same brand as the product in the advertisement? _(Answers will vary.)_____________________________

____

____

12. Would this advertisement affect your interest in using any of the other products made by this brand? Explain why or why not. _(Answers will vary.)________________________

____

Your Food Habits

Activity C   Name ____

Chapter 1   Date _________________________   Period_______________________

Answer the following questions about your food habits in the space provided.

1. How many meals do you eat each day? _(Answers will vary.)_________________

2. How many snacks do you eat each day? _(Answers will vary.)_______________

3. What size portions do you eat? _(Answers will vary.)____________________

4. How often do you take second helpings? _(Answers will vary.)_____________

5. How much time do you spend at each meal? _(Answers will vary.)___________

6. At what times do you eat each day? _(Answers will vary.)_________________

7. Is your eating behavior different on weekends than it is on weekdays? If so, explain how and why.
   _(Answers will vary.)____

   ____

   ____

8. Where do you do most of your eating? _(Answers will vary.)_______________

9. With whom do you do most of your eating? _(Answers will vary.)___________

10. What factors, other than hunger, sometimes cause you to eat? _(Answers will vary.)___

   ____

11. What else, if anything, do you do while you are eating? _(Answers will vary.)___

12. How does food make you feel? _(Answers will vary.)_____________________

13. What do you grab to satisfy hunger in a hurry? _(Answers will vary.)______

14. What is your favorite food? _(Answers will vary.)______________________

15. Name a food you do not like and explain why you do not like it. _(Answers will vary.)___

   ____

16. How does culture affect your food habits? _(Answers will vary.)__________

   ____

17. How does your lifestyle affect your food habits? _(Answers will vary.)_____

   ____

18. How do family members and friends affect your food habits? _(Answers will vary.)___

   ____

19. How does mass media affect your food habits? _(Answers will vary.)_______

   ____

20. How do current trends affect your food habits? _(Answers will vary.)______

   ____

The Food Supply

Activity D   Name ____

Chapter 1   Date ______________________   Period__________________________

Identify which of the listed factors that affect the food supply is represented by each of the following statements. Write the letter of the correct response in the space provided to the left of each number.

____E____ 1. Chow bought tofu in an aseptic package designed to keep the unopened tofu fresh for months.

____C____ 2. The Nutrition Facts panel required on each package of Darnell's favorite breakfast cereal helps him find out how much fiber a serving provides.

____B____ 3. Janine had to go to an Asian market in the city to get the Thai chili paste her recipe required.

____A____ 4. Jason is disappointed at the cost of peaches this year because a late frost destroyed a large portion of the crop.

____C____ 5. Jeff notices the package of chicken he picks up has a stamp indicating the poultry is federally inspected.

____E____ 6. Latrise buys yogurt sweetened with a new artificial sweetener as a low-calorie, nutritious snack.

____B____ 7. Pedro is a Colombian coffee bean harvester who can barely afford corn and potatoes to feed his family.

____A____ 8. Ray is a Midwestern soybean farmer who irrigates his fields to ensure the plants receive an adequate amount of water.

____D____ 9. Shantal has no refrigerator in her rural African home, so she gathers fruits and vegetables from her garden each day to make her meals.

____E____ 10. Susan ordered seeds for a new variety of tomatoes that are supposed to grow bigger and ripen faster than other tomatoes.

____D____ 11. The locally grown apples at Carla's Michigan supermarket are a bargain in the fall.

____D____ 12. Vicki's aunt in Wisconsin pays more for Texas grapefruit than Vicki's mom pays in their local San Antonio supermarket.

____C____ 13. A news report stated Farm Fresh apple cider had been recalled because federal inspectors found samples in the processing plant to be contaminated.

____A____ 14. David noticed his crop yields were always highest in the fields along the riverbanks, where the soil was richest.

____B____ 15. Workers from a hunger-relief organization taught people in Muhundi's village how to rotate crops and fertilize with compost to improve their crop yields.

A. environment
B. economics
C. government
D. regional agriculture
E. technology

Nutritional Needs

Nutrition Facts

Activity A   Name ____

Chapter 2   Date ____________________________ Period ______________

After researching or discussing the various nutrients, list their function(s) and food sources in the chart.
Then answer the questions that follow.

Nutrient	Function(s)	Food Sources
Carbohydrates	(Chart answers will vary.)	
Fats		
Proteins		
Vitamin A		
Vitamin D		
Vitamin E		
Vitamin K		
Vitamin C		
Thiamin		
Riboflavin		
Niacin		
Vitamin B_6		
Folate		
Vitamin B_{12}		
Pantothenic acid		
Biotin		
Calcium		
Phosphorus		
Magnesium		
Sodium		
Chloride		
Potassium		

(Continued)

Nutrient	Function(s)	Food Sources
Iron		
Zinc		
Iodine		
Fluoride		
Water		

1. Do you regularly eat sources of each of the nutrients listed in this chart? (Answers will vary.) ________

   ____

2. If you answered *no* to the above question, which nutrients are lacking in your diet? ________________
   (Answers will vary.) ____

   ____

3. Why is it necessary to include sources of each of these nutrients in your diet? (Answers will vary.) ____

   ____

   ____

4. How can this chart serve as a guide in choosing the foods you eat? (Answers will vary.) ____________

   ____

   ____

5. How would you define good nutrition? (Answers will vary.) ____________________________________

   ____

   ____

Nutrient Deficiencies and Excesses

Activity B Name ____________________

Chapter 2 Date ____________________ Period __________

Match the following nutrient deficiencies and excesses on the left with the descriptions of their symptoms on the right. Beneath each item, check the minus (–) box if the condition is caused by a nutrient deficiency. Check the plus (+) box if the condition is caused by a nutrient excess. Then write the name of the nutrient related to the condition in the blank.

__H__ 1. PEM
– ☑ + ☐ protein ____________________

__B__ 2. night blindness
– ☑ + ☐ vitamin A ____________________

__K__ 3. rickets
– ☑ + ☐ vitamin D ____________________

__F__ 4. scurvy
– ☑ + ☐ vitamin C ____________________

__A__ 5. beriberi
– ☑ + ☐ thiamin ____________________

__E__ 6. pellagra
– ☑ + ☐ niacin ____________________

__I__ 7. pernicious anemia
– ☑ + ☐ vitamin B_{12} ____________________

__G__ 8. osteoporosis
– ☑ + ☐ calcium ____________________

__D__ 9. hypertension
– ☐ + ☑ sodium ____________________

__C__ 10. goiter
– ☑ + ☐ iodine ____________________

A. numbness in feet and ankles followed by cramping pains and stiffness in legs

B. reduced ability to see in dim light

C. enlargement of the thyroid gland

D. high blood pressure

E. skin lesions, digestive problems, mental disorders, death

F. weakness, bleeding gums, loss of teeth, and internal bleeding

G. porous, brittle bones

H. fatigue and weight loss in adults; diarrhea, infections, and stunted growth in children

I. abnormally large red blood cells, depression, and drowsiness

J. swelling caused by buildup of fluids

K. crooked legs, misshapen breastbone

Nutrition Crossword

Name ___________________________

Date _______________________   Period _____________

(Continued)

Down

1. High blood pressure.
2. The study of how the body uses the nutrients in foods that are eaten.
4. Starches and fiber are often called ______ carbohydrates.
6. A condition resulting from a calcium deficiency, which is characterized by porous, brittle bones.
7. A vitamin that dissolves in fats and can be stored in the fatty tissues of the body.
8. A mineral, such as iron or iodine, that is needed in the diet in amounts less than 100 milligrams per day is called a(n) ______ element.
11. A condition resulting from deficiencies of various nutrients, which is characterized by a reduced number of red blood cells in the bloodstream.
12. A nutrient required by the body to lubricate the joints and body cells and help regulate body temperature.
13. The bodily process of breaking food down into simpler compounds the body can use.
14. A disease of the nervous system resulting from a thiamin deficiency.
16. A chemical chain containing carbon, hydrogen, and oxygen atoms that is the basic component of all lipids.
19. One of the six basic types of nutrients that is required for growth, repair, and maintenance of every body cell.
20. A disease resulting from a niacin deficiency.
21. One of the six basic types of nutrients that is the body's chief source of energy.
22. A fatlike substance that occurs only in foods of animal origin.
25. A protein containing all nine essential amino acids in sufficient amounts.
26. A disease resulting from a vitamin D deficiency.
27. A fatty acid with an odd molecular shape that is created in hydrogenated oils.
28. A form of sugar carried in the bloodstream for energy use throughout the body.
30. A condition resulting from a vitamin A deficiency is called ______ blindness.

Across

1. A process used to turn liquid oils into more highly saturated solid fats.
3. The chemical processes that take place in the cells after the body absorbs nutrients.
5. An illness caused by the lack of a sufficient amount of a nutrient is called a ______ disease.
9. A type of fatty acid that is missing one hydrogen atom.
10. A mucus- and enzyme-containing liquid secreted by the mouth.
15. One of 20 types of small units that make up proteins is a(n) ______ acid.
17. A form of complex carbohydrate from plants that humans cannot digest.
18. One of the six basic types of nutrients that are important energy sources.
19. Waves of contractions of the muscular walls of the digestive tract, which push food through the tract.
23. One of the six basic nutrient types that is an inorganic substance and becomes part of the bones, soft tissues, and body fluids.
24. One of the six basic types of nutrients that is a complex organic substance needed in small amounts for normal growth, maintenance, and reproduction.
29. A disease resulting from a vitamin C deficiency.
31. A chemical substance from food the body needs to live.
32. The process of taking nutrients into the body and making them part of the body.
33. A condition that may result if the diet does not contain enough protein and calories.
34. A visible enlargement of the thyroid gland resulting from an iodine deficiency.

How the Body Uses Food

Activity D   Name _______________________________________

Chapter 2   Date ___________________________   Period ____________

Answer the following questions related to energy needs and the processes of digestion, absorption, and metabolism.

1. Describe the digestive tract. The digestive tract is a tube about 30 feet long that extends from the mouth to the anus and includes the esophagus, stomach, small intestine, and large intestine.

2. What are the two phases of the digestive process? the mechanical phase and the chemical phase

3. What is peristalsis? Peristalsis is waves of contractions of the muscular walls of the digestive tract, which push food through the tract.

4. What enzyme-containing fluid is secreted by the stomach? gastric juices

5. What role do enzymes play in the process of digestion? Digestive enzymes help break down carbohydrates, proteins, and fats into simple substances the body can absorb and use.

6. Place numbers in the blanks to indicate the order in which the following nutrients leave the stomach during digestion.

   __2__ proteins   __3__ fats   __1__ carbohydrates

7. If you were to choose one of the foods in the following table for a snack, which one would satisfy your hunger the longest? Explain your answer.

Food	Protein	Fat	Carbohydrate
1-inch cube Cheddar cheese	4 grams	6 grams	trace
apple	trace	trace	21 grams
roasted chicken drumstick	12 grams	2 grams	0 grams

   The cheese would satisfy hunger longest because it has the highest fat content. Fats stay in the stomach longer than carbohydrates or proteins.

8. Where does most absorption take place? in the small intestine

9. What are villi and what role do they play in the process of absorption? Villi are hairlike fingers that line the small intestine and increase its absorptive surface by more than 600 percent.

10. Where do metabolic reactions take place? within the cells

11. Give an example of how each of the following nutrients could be used as a result of metabolic reactions.

   Carbohydrates: used for energy, converted to glycogen, stored as fat

   Fats: used for fuel

   Proteins: used for cell maintenance; used for cell growth; used for the synthesis of enzymes, antibodies, and nonessential amino acids; used as an energy source

Making Healthful Choices

Choosing to Change

Activity A   Name _______________________________________

Chapter 3   Date _______________________   Period ____________

Read the scenarios and answer the questions that follow in the space provided.

1. Danny's career and social life keep him too busy to spend much time shopping for and preparing nutritious foods. He often chooses to skip breakfast, grab burgers and fries for lunch, and meet friends for pizza after work. Danny seldom chooses to eat fruits, vegetables, whole grains, or dairy foods. What are some possible health risks associated with Danny's food choices? _______________

   (Answers will vary.) ____

   What changes could Danny choose that would make his food choices more healthful? _____________

   (Answers will vary.) ____

2. Amondi's downtown apartment is just eight blocks from the office building where she works. Each day, she chooses to take the bus to and from work. Amondi chooses to spend her evenings chatting with friends on the phone, updating her page on a social networking website, or watching television. Amondi often chooses to spend her weekends curled up with a book or having friends over to talk or play cards. What are some possible health risks associated with Amondi's activity choices? _________

   (Answers will vary.) ____

   What changes could Amondi choose that would make her activity choices more healthful? _________

   (Answers will vary.) ____

3. Park does not choose to smoke, but many of his coworkers do. Each day, Park chooses to eat lunch with his coworkers in an area where they are permitted to smoke. What are some possible health risks associated with Park's lifestyle choices involving tobacco? _____________________________

   (Answers will vary.) ____

   What changes could Park choose that would make his lifestyle choices more healthful?____________

   (Answers will vary.) ____

4. Mariana and her friends are known for always being ready to have a wild and crazy time. They might choose to go out after work, dancing on Saturday night, or tailgating on Sunday afternoon. No matter what activities they choose, however, Mariana and her friends frequently choose to drink excessive amounts of alcohol. What are some possible health risks associated with Mariana and her friends' lifestyle choices involving alcohol? ____

   (Answers will vary.) ____

   What changes could Mariana and her friends choose that would make their lifestyle choices more healthful? ____

   (Answers will vary.) ____

Promoting the Dietary Guidelines

Name ______________________________

Date ______________________   Period __________

Suppose you work for a public relations company that has been contracted by the USDA. You are assigned to design various kitchen-related items that will help promote the Dietary Guidelines for Americans. To prepare your proposal, use color, illustrations, and artistic typefaces to emphasize four of the following consumer messages and action steps on the items pictured below. (Answers will vary.)

Balance calories.
- Enjoy your food, but eat less.
- Avoid oversized portions.

Eat more of some foods.
- Make half your plate fruits and vegetables.
- Switch to fat-free or low-fat (1%) milk.

Eat less of some foods.
- Compare sodium in foods like soup, bread, and frozen meals—and choose the foods with lower numbers.
- Drink water instead of sugary drinks.

refrigerator magnet

shopping list pad

rubber jar opener

bag clip

Eating from MyPlate

Activity C   **Name** ___________________________________

Chapter 3   **Date** ___________________________ **Period** _____________

Answer the following questions about the MyPlate food groups. Write your responses in the space provided.

1. What are your two favorite foods from each of the subgroups in the grains group?

    A. whole grains _(Answers will vary.)____________________________________

    B. refined grains _(Answers will vary.)__________________________________

2. Why is it recommended that people make at least half their daily grains group choices from the whole grains subgroup?

    Whole-grain foods are high in fiber._________________________________

3. What is your favorite vegetable in each of the following subgroups?

    A. dark green vegetables _(Answers will vary.)___________________________

    B. red and orange vegetables _(Answers will vary.)_______________________

    C. beans and peas _(Answers will vary.)_________________________________

    D. starchy vegetables _(Answers will vary.)______________________________

    E. other vegetables _(Answers will vary.)________________________________

4. What nutrients are supplied by the vegetable group? ____________________________

    Vegetables are good sources of vitamins, minerals, and fiber.__________

5. What are your three favorite foods from the fruit group? _(Answers will vary.)__________

    ____

6. What forms of fruits are included in the fruit group?_____________________________

    The fruit group includes fresh, canned, frozen, and dried fruits and pure (100%) fruit juices.

7. What are your three favorite foods from the dairy group? _(Answers will vary.)__________

    ____

8. Foods from the dairy group are the best sources of what nutrient? calcium____________

9. What are your three favorite foods from the protein foods group? _(Answers will vary.)____

    ____

10. Foods from the protein foods group are excellent sources of what nutrient? protein______

11. What foods do you choose that contribute small amounts of oils to your diet? _(Answers will vary.)___

    ____

12. Why should people consume only small amounts of foods that provide mostly solid fats and/or added sugars?

    Foods that are high in solid fats and/or added sugars are often high in calories. They also tend to be low in vitamins and minerals._________________________________

Choosing Wisely When Shopping

Name _______________________________________

Date _____________________________ **Period** _____________

Read the following statements about purchasing food. Circle *T* if the statement is true and circle *F* if the statement is false.

(T) F 1. Processing often decreases the nutritional value of foods.

(T) F 2. Fresh foods should be used as soon after purchase as possible.

T (F) 3. Most canned vegetables are lower in sodium than fresh vegetables.

T (F) 4. Fruit juices are higher in fiber than fresh fruits.

(T) F 5. Beef round steak and pork tenderloin are lean cuts of meat.

T (F) 6. Dark meat pieces of chicken and turkey are lower in fat than light meat pieces.

(T) F 7. Most varieties of fresh fish and shellfish are low in fat.

(T) F 8. A portion that is larger than the stated serving size will provide more than the stated amounts of calories and nutrients.

T (F) 9. Any food providing more than 200 calories per serving is considered high in calories.

T (F) 10. A percent Daily Value of 20 percent or less is considered low for a given nutrient.

(T) F 11. Beef fat in an ingredient list is a source of added saturated fats.

(T) F 12. Nutritional labeling can help you compare similar products and different brands of the same product.

T (F) 13. English muffins are a good source of complex carbohydrates, but they are also high in fat.

(T) F 14. Although many breakfast cereals are good sources of fiber, some are high in added sugar and sodium.

T (F) 15. Instant hot cereals tend to be much lower in sodium than regular and quick-cooking products.

(T) F 16. Fruits canned in juice are lower in sugar than those canned in syrup.

(T) F 17. Some fruit drinks and fruit punches contain very little fruit juice.

(T) F 18. Beans, peas, and lentils are low-fat, high-fiber meat alternates.

T (F) 19. Most processed meats, like luncheon meats and hot dogs, are low in fat but high in sodium.

(T) F 20. Fish canned in water is lower in fat than fish canned in oil.

(T) F 21. Many soups, sauce mixes, and packaged entrees are high in sodium.

T (F) 22. Stick margarine is a good choice for a product low in trans fatty acids.

(T) F 23. Many refined grain products, such as cakes and cookies, are also high in solid fats and added sugars.

T (F) 24. Wheat flour is a whole-grain ingredient.

Preparing Healthful Food

Activity E   **Name** ____

Chapter 3   **Date** ___________________________   **Period** ____________

Answer the following questions about preparing foods based on the Dietary Guidelines for Americans. Write your answers in the space provided.

1. What is the advantage of preparing foods from scratch?

   Preparing foods from scratch gives you more control over the amount of added fat, sugars, and salt.

2. How large is a 3-ounce (84 g) portion of meat, poultry, or fish?

   A 3-ounce (84 g) portion of protein food is about the size of a deck of playing cards.

3. How should meat and poultry be prepared before cooking? ___________________________

   Trim all visible fat from the meat. Remove skin from the poultry.

4. What is the value of actually measuring out servings of some favorite foods?

   Observing what serving sizes look like in your tableware will help you serve appropriate portions and avoid exceeding calorie needs.

5. How can you reduce the fat when preparing packaged pasta, rice, stuffing, and sauce mixes?

   Using only half the amount of butter or margarine suggested on packages will help reduce fat when preparing packaged pasta, rice, stuffing, and sauce mixes.

6. What can you do to reduce the fat added by such toppings as salad dressings, mayonnaise, sour cream, and cream cheese?

   Salad dressings, mayonnaise, sour cream, and cream cheese should be used sparingly, or try reduced-fat versions or plain nonfat yogurt in place of these products.

7. How can you limit your sodium and fat intake when preparing vegetables? ___________________

   Vegetables can be flavored with herbs and lemon juice instead of salt and butter.

8. What modifications should be made to a recipe calling for cheese or condensed soup?

   Salt can be omitted from recipes calling for other sodium-containing ingredients, such as cheese or condensed soup.

9. What other modifications might you make to a cake recipe in which you wanted to reduce the sugar?

   Adding vanilla or spices, such as cinnamon, ginger, or cloves, makes recipes for baked goods seem sweeter when the amount of sugar in the recipes has been reduced.

10. How can you prepare egg dishes, such as omelets and scrambled eggs, while still limiting your cholesterol intake?

    Portions of omelets and scrambled eggs can be stretched by adding extra egg whites in place of whole eggs, which contain high-cholesterol yolks.

Dining Habits Survey

Activity F   **Name** ____

Chapter 3   **Date** _______________________   **Period** ____________

Survey five teens about their habits and preferences when dining out. Record their answers in the table provided. Then use your survey findings to make a general recommendation for teens regarding their food choices when eating out. *(Table answers will vary.)*

1. What is your gender?   A. male B. female

2. How often do you eat away from home?   A. less than once a week B. once a week C. two to three times a week D. four to five times a week E. once a day F. more than once a day

3. Where do you most often get the food you eat away from home?   A. fast-food restaurants B. school cafeteria C. sit-down restaurants D. pizza parlors and/or sandwich shops E. snack bars and concession stands F. vending machines G convenience or grocery stores H. friends' homes

4. What types of foods do you most often choose when you eat away from home?   A. hamburgers and other sandwiches B. pizza C. chips and other salty snacks D. fried foods E. candy, ice cream, desserts, or other sweets F. soft drinks and shakes

5. What impact does nutritional value have on your food choices when eating out?   A. a great deal of impact B. some impact C. little impact D. no impact

6. Who do you usually eat with when you eat away from home?   A. family members B. friends C. dating partner D. coworkers E. usually eat alone

7. Why do you usually eat away from home?   A. convenience B. entertainment C. variety D. to be with friends E. to avoid cooking F. habit

8. What factor has the greatest influence on the foods you choose?   A. cost B. personal likes and dislikes C. nutrition D. choices of people eating with me

Survey Responses

Question	Person 1	Person 2	Person 3	Person 4	Person 5
1.					
2.					
3.					
4.					
5.					
6.					
7.					
8.					

What conclusions can you draw from your survey findings? *(Answers will vary.)* ______________

____

____

What recommendation would you make to teens about their food choices when eating out based on these conclusions? *(Answers will vary.)* ________________________________

____

Nutrition and Fitness Through the Life Span

Baby Food

Activity A **Name** _______________________________

Chapter 4 **Date** _____________________ **Period** __________

Interview the mother of an infant. Record her responses to the questions that follow in the space provided.

1. How much weight did you gain during your pregnancy? __(Answers will vary.)__

2. Was your weight gain within your obstetrician's recommendations? __(Answers will vary.)__

3. What changes did you make in your diet when you were pregnant? __(Answers will vary.)__
____

4. What, if any, dietary supplements did your obstetrician prescribe during your pregnancy? ________
(Answers will vary.)

5. How old is your baby? __(Answers will vary.)__

6. How much did your child weigh at birth? __(Answers will vary.)__
How much does your child weigh now? __(Answers will vary.)__
What is the weight increase or decrease? __(Answers will vary.)__

7. How long was your child at birth? __(Answers will vary.)__
How long is your child now? __(Answers will vary.)__
What is the length increase? __(Answers will vary.)__

8. Is your baby breast-fed or formula-fed? __(Answers will vary.)__

9. How many times a day do you feed your baby? __(Answers will vary.)__

10. What, if anything, do you feed your baby besides breast milk or formula? __(Answers will vary.)__
____

11. How much milk and solid food does your baby consume each day? __(Answers will vary.)__
____

12. What, if any, dietary supplements has your pediatrician recommended for your baby? __________
(Answers will vary.)

13. When did you, or at what age do you plan to, introduce solid foods into your baby's diet? __________
(Answers will vary.)

14. What solid foods did or will you introduce first? __(Answers will vary.)__
____

15. What procedure has your pediatrician recommended for introducing new foods to your baby? ______
(Answers will vary.)

Diets in the Life Cycle

Activity B   **Name** ____

Chapter 4   **Date** _______________________   **Period** ____________

Answer the questions related to changing dietary needs throughout the life cycle based on the menus that follow. Write your responses in the space provided.

Breakfast

2 slices	French toast with 1 tablespoon (15 mL) syrup	½ cup (125 mL)	Orange juice
		1 cup (250 mL)	Coffee

Lunch

1 cup (250 mL)	Chili [made with 2 ounces cooked ground beef, ½ cup (125 mL) kidney beans, ½ cup (125 mL) corn]	2 slices	Whole-wheat bread
		½ cup (125 mL)	Canned peaches
		1 cup (250 mL)	Low-fat milk

Dinner

3 ounces (84 g)	Ham		Small green salad with 1 tablespoon (15 mL) French dressing
1 square	Cornbread with 1 teaspoon (5 mL) margarine	1 slice	Cheesecake
½ cup (125 mL)	Carrots	1 cup (250 mL)	Low-fat milk

1. How might a pregnant woman modify these menus to meet her special nutritional needs?
   (Answers will vary.)

2. What foods could you substitute in this lunch menu that would appeal more to a preschooler? Explain your answer.____
   (Answers will vary.)

3. What foods could you substitute in this breakfast menu that would appeal to a school-age child who does not like traditional breakfast foods? ____
   (Answers will vary.)

4. Consider the amounts from each food group recommended for an active teen girl who needs 2,400 calories per day. How could you adjust portion sizes and/or add snack foods to these menus to meet these increased nutritional needs?____
   (Answers will vary.)

5. What foods could you substitute in these menus to meet the calcium needs of an older adult who does not like to drink milk? ____
   (Answers will vary.)

6. What foods could you substitute in these menus to meet the protein needs of a lacto-ovo vegetarian?
   (Answers will vary.)

Nutrition Advice

Activity C **Name** _______________________________________

Chapter 4 **Date** _____________________________ **Period** ____________

Imagine that you write a column called *The Diet Counselor* for a local newspaper. Use chapter information to answer the following letters from your readers about their nutrition concerns. Write your responses in the space provided.

Dear Diet Counselor,

Since learning last week that my wife is pregnant, I've been cooking up a storm. I've been making big breakfasts, big lunches, big dinners, and big snacks. Despite my efforts, she's eating no more now than she did before getting pregnant. I'm afraid she's not getting enough nutrients for the baby. Please advise.

Expectant Father

1. Dear Dad,

   (Answers will vary.)

   ____

   ____

   ____

   ____

   ____

   D.C.

Dear Diet Counselor,

My three-year-old son is a finicky eater. At some meals, he barely eats at all. Should I be concerned?

Muddled Mom

3. Dear Muddled,

   (Answers will vary.)

   ____

   ____

   ____

   ____

   ____

   D.C.

Dear Diet Counselor,

My sister has been feeding my newborn nephew about eight times a day. Isn't feeding him so often going to cause him to become fat?

A Doting Aunt

2. Dear Auntie,

   (Answers will vary.)

   ____

   ____

   ____

   ____

   ____

   D.C.

Dear Diet Counselor,

After my parents leave for work, I'm in charge of getting my nine-year-old brother off to school. He doesn't really like cereal and toast, so most mornings he just skips breakfast. Is this okay?

Big Brother

4. Dear Bro,

   (Answers will vary.)

   ____

   ____

   ____

   ____

   ____

   D.C.

(Continued)

Dear Diet Counselor,

I'm 15 years old and I'm about 20 pounds over-weight. I'm thinking about trying the "Squeeze Yourself Thin—All Lemon and Grapefruit Juice Diet." Even though she has a friend who lost 37 pounds on this diet, my mom's been trying to talk me out of trying it. What can I say to convince her?

Heavy Teen

5. Dear H.T.,

(Answers will vary.)

____

____

____

____

____

____

D.C.

Dear Diet Counselor,

My job, family, and community activities keep me pretty busy. I find myself relying on fast-food restaurants for many of my meals. As a result, I've started to put on a little unwanted weight. What can I do to improve my diet?

Middle-Aged Bulge

6. Dear Bulge,

(Answers will vary.)

____

____

____

____

____

____

D.C.

Dear Diet Counselor,

My grandmother's doctor told her she has brittle bones due to a poor diet. Is there something my grandmother could eat to make her bones stronger? Will I suffer from brittle bones when I am her age?

A Concerned Granddaughter

7. Dear Concerned,

(Answers will vary.)

____

____

____

____

____

____

D.C.

Dear Diet Counselor,

One of my friends told me he is a "lacto-ovo" vegetarian. What does this mean?

A Meat Lover

8. Dear Meat Lover,

(Answers will vary.)

____

____

____

____

____

____

D.C.

Life Span Fitness

Activity D Name ____

Chapter 4 Date ______________________________ Period ____________

Put yourself in the role of a recreation director at a local community center. One of your tasks is to plan a variety of fitness classes to meet the needs of people in your community at all stages of the life span. Your center has an indoor track and space for exercise classes, basketball, and volleyball. It also has an outdoor playground, ball diamond, and soccer field. You can use any of the facilities at the center as you plan your classes. Write descriptions to go with each of the following class titles for a brochure the center is printing about their upcoming programs.

1. **Motherhood in Motion** *(pregnant women)*
   (Answers will vary.)

2. **New Mommy Makeover** *(women 6 weeks to 6 months after giving birth)*
   (Answers will vary.)

3. **Build Up Your Baby** *(parents and children up to 18 months)*
   (Answers will vary.)

4. **Rug Rat Runaround** *(parents and walking children up to age 6)*
   (Answers will vary.)

5. **Keep Fit Kids Klub** *(children ages 6 to 12)*
   (Answers will vary.)

6. **Viral Vitality** *(teens)*
   (Answers will vary.)

7. **After-Work Workout** *(adults)*
   (Answers will vary.)

8. **Senior Sweat Session** *(older adults)*
   (Answers will vary.)

Food Assistance Programs

Activity E   **Name** ___________________________________

Chapter 4   **Date** _____________________   **Period** ___________

Assume you are a social worker employed by a state agency to help people enroll in food assistance programs. You have reviewed the eligibility forms of each of the following applicants and determined they meet the requirements to receive program benefits. Your next step is to fill out the approval forms for the appropriate assistance programs. For each applicant described below, place a checkmark on your case files in the appropriate boxes to indicate which approval form(s) you will complete: WIC (Women, Infants, and Children), *NSLP/SBP/SFSP* (National School Lunch Program/School Breakfast Program/Summer Food Service Program), *SNAP* (Supplemental Nutrition Assistance Program), and/or *Elderly NP* (Elderly Nutrition Program).

Decker, Amy

Forms completed: ☑ **WIC**   ☑ **NSLP/SBP/SFSP**   ☐ **SNAP**   ☐ **Elderly NP**

Case notes: *16-year-old mother, enrolled at Crestville H.S. Daughter, Kaylie, is 4 months old.*

Decker, Kaylie

Forms completed: ☑ **WIC**   ☐ **NSLP/SBP/SFSP**   ☐ **SNAP**   ☐ **Elderly NP**

Case notes: *4-month-old female in care of teen mother, Amy.*

Grayson, Ida Mae

Forms completed: ☐ **WIC**   ☐ **NSLP/SBP/SFSP**   ☐ **SNAP**   ☑ **Elderly NP**

Case notes: *67-year-old female, uses wheelchair, has no available transportation. Income not eligible for SNAP.*

Phillips, Trevor

Forms completed: ☐ **WIC**   ☑ **NSLP/SBP/SFSP**   ☐ **SNAP**   ☐ **Elderly NP**

Case notes: *10-year-old male in care of grandmother, Virginia Milton. Currently attends Rosehill Elementary School.*

Stanton, Carla

Forms completed: ☑ **WIC**   ☐ **NSLP/SBP/SFSP**   ☐ **SNAP**   ☐ **Elderly NP**

Case notes: *23-year-old female, pregnant, employed part-time in minimum wage position. Husband, Duane, currently unemployed.*

Wheeler, Charles

Forms completed: ☐ **WIC**   ☐ **NSLP/SBP/SFSP**   ☑ **SNAP**   ☐ **Elderly NP**

Case notes: *27-year-old male, underemployed, supports 3 school-age children.*

Staying Active and Managing Weight

Your Energy Needs

Activity A   **Name** _______________________________________

Chapter 5   **Date** ______________________________ **Period** _____________

Complete the following items about the body's energy needs. Write your responses in the space provided.

1. What are four functions for which the human body requires energy? ___________________________
   move, produce heat, carry on internal processes, support growth and repair

In each of the following pairs, place a check beside the description of the person who is likely to have the higher basal metabolic rate. In the space below each pair, explain the reason for your choice.

2. _____ A. 5'10" tall person   ✓ B. 6'1" tall person
   A tall person has a larger body surface area than a short person.

3. ✓ A. male   _____ B. female
   Men usually have a larger amount of lean muscle tissue than women.

4. ✓ A. 15-year-old   _____ B. 30-year-old
   Adolescents have a higher basal metabolism than adults because they are in a period of rapid growth.

5. _____ A. a person with a body temperature of 98.6°F
   ✓ B. a person with a body temperature of 101.2°F
   An increase in body temperature increases basal metabolism.

In each of the following pairs, choose the one that will require more energy. In the space below each pair, explain the reason for your choice.

6. _____ A. bicycling at 8 miles per hour   ✓ B. bicycling at 12 miles per hour
   A more intense task requires more energy.

7. ✓ A. a 195-pound man jogging at 6 miles per hour
   _____ B. a 150-pound man jogging at 6 miles per hour
   A larger body size uses more energy than a smaller body size to do the same task.

8. _____ A. typing a letter   ✓ B. vacuuming a floor
   A more intense task requires more energy.

9. ✓ A. mowing the lawn when it is 85°F outside   _____ B. mowing the lawn when it is 72°F outside
   It takes more energy to do a task in a warmer environment.

10. Indicate how body weight is affected by energy intake from foods by writing *increase*, *decrease*, or *remain the same* after each of the following equations.

    A. energy intake > energy expended *increase*

    B. energy intake = energy expended *remain the same*

    C. energy intake < energy expended *decrease*

11. How many calories make up 1 pound of body weight? *3,500*

12. What unit do food scientists use to measure the energy value of foods? *kilocalorie*

Being Physically Active

Activity B Name ____

Chapter 5 Date _____________________________ Period _____________

Answer the following questions to help you analyze your current level of physical activity and make plans for increasing your level of activity. Write your answers in the space provided.

1. Rank how important each of the benefits of physical activity are to you, with 1 being the most important and 8 being the least important. (Answers will vary.)

   _______________ builds strong bones

   _______________ contributes to overall fitness

   _______________ helps burn calories, aiding in weight maintenance

   _______________ improves self-esteem

   _______________ keeps skin healthy

   _______________ provides fun social outlet

   _______________ reduces risk of some chronic diseases

   _______________ tones muscles

2. How much time do you currently spend being physically active each day? (Answers will vary.) ____________

3. How could you make more time in your schedule to increase your level of physical activity? ________
   (Answers will vary.) ____

4. In what types of physical activities that improve flexibility do you currently participate? ____________
   (Answers will vary.) ____

5. In what types of physical activities that improve strength do you currently participate? ____________
   (Answers will vary.) ____

6. In what types of physical activities that improve balance do you currently participate?____________
   (Answers will vary.) ____

7. In what types of physical activities that improve endurance do you currently participate? __________
   (Answers will vary.) ____

8. What is the next physical activity goal you would like to try to reach? (Answers will vary.) __________

   ____

9. What types of activity do you most enjoy? (Answers will vary.) ________________________________

   ____

10. What factors are most likely to keep you from being physically active? (Answers will vary.) __________

    ____

11. What can you do to overcome these factors? (Answers will vary.) ______________________________

    ____

12. With whom do you engage in physical fitness activities? (Answers will vary.) ____________________

    ____

The Sports Nutritionist

Activity C   Name ____

Chapter 5   Date _______________________________ Period ______________

Presume you are a registered dietitian who counsels teen athletes to help them maximize their athletic performance. Read the client files that follow and write your recommendations for each situation in the space provided. (Answers will vary.)

Client name   **Glen Walker**
Age **17**   Height **5′1″**   Weight **167**
Sport **Track—1,600 m**

Concerns
Toward the ends of his races, Glen often gets headaches. He becomes dizzy and confused and his pace drops off dramatically.

Recommendations

____

____

____

____

____

____

Client name   **Keiko Hoshi**
Age **14**   Height **4′11″**   Weight **93**
Sport   **Gymnastics**

Concerns
Keiko is very concerned about keeping her weight down for competition. She seldom consumes more than 2 meal shakes and a salad each day.

Recommendations

____

____

____

____

____

____

Client name   **Gerald Toliver**
Age **18**   Height **6′2″**   Weight **221**
Sport   **Football—defensive tackle**

Concerns
Gerald wants to be sure he's eating the best diet for energy and performance. He is considering taking protein supplements to help increase muscle mass.

Recommendations

____

____

____

____

____

____

Client name   **Christi Davis**
Age **16**   Height **5′8″**   Weight **133**
Sport   **Volleyball**

Concerns
Christi wants to know when and what to eat before a game so she'll have maximum energy and won't get stomach cramps.

Recommendations

____

____

____

____

____

____

Making a Weight Management Plan

Activity D Name _______________________________

Chapter 5 Date ____________________________ Period ____________

Analyze the menus that follow and consider how you would alter them to help an adult lose weight. Then complete this activity following the steps.

	Calories	Fat (g)
Breakfast		
1. Orange juice from concentrate, ¾ cup (175 mL)	83	0
2. Granola, 1 ounce (28 g)	125	5
3. Whole milk, ½ cup (125 mL)	75	4
4. Coffee, with sugar	15	0
Lunch		
5. Oil pack tuna, 3 ounces (84 g)	165	7
6. White bread, 2 slices (18 per loaf)	130	2
7. Tossed salad greens, 1 cup (250 mL)	5	0
8. Thousand Island dressing, 1 tablespoon (15 mL)	60	6
9. Whole milk, 1 cup (250 mL)	150	8
10. Chocolate chip cookies, 4 medium	180	9
Dinner		
11. Broiled steak, 3 ounces (84 g)	240	15
12. Baked potato, 1 medium with skin	220	0
13. Sour cream, 1 tablespoon (15 mL)	25	3
14. Steamed broccoli, ½ cup (125 mL)	23	0
15. Cheese sauce, 2 tablespoons (30 mL)	38	2
16. Dinner roll, 1 small	85	2
17. Butter, 1 teaspoon (5 mL)	35	4
18. Vanilla ice cream, 1 cup (250 mL)	270	14
19. Iced tea, with sugar	30	0
Snack		
20. Chocolate bar with almonds, 2 ounces (60 g)	300	20
Total	**2254**	**105**

1. In the first, second, third, and fourth columns of the table on the next page, list the item number, name, calorie value, and fat value of each food you would eliminate or replace in the menus above.

2. In the fifth column, list foods you would substitute opposite those you are replacing. Leave this column blank opposite foods you are eliminating. (When selecting substitutes, remember to choose foods of similar or greater nutritive value than those you are replacing. Be sure to include the recommended daily amounts from each food group in your adapted menus.)

3. Use the Food-A-Pedia interactive tool at the USDA SuperTracker website to determine the calorie and fat values of the foods you are substituting. List those values in the last two columns.

4. Compute the total calorie and fat savings.

5. Answer the questions that follow the table.

(Continued)

Item Number	Food Being Replaced or Eliminated	Calorie Value	Fat Value	Substitute Food	Calorie Value	Fat Value
	(Table answers will vary.)					

Total calories of replaced or eliminated foods   (Answers will vary.)

Total calories of substitute foods   (Answers will vary.)

Total calorie savings   (Answers will vary.)

Total grams of fat in replaced or eliminated foods   (Answers will vary.)

Total grams of fat in substitute foods   (Answers will vary.)

Total grams of fat saved   (Answers will vary.)

1. Identify five hazards of obesity. ____________________________
   (List five:) early death; more likely to suffer from hypertension; more likely to suffer from heart ailments; more likely to suffer from cancer; higher insurance rates; strain on bones, muscles, and organs; more effort needed to walk, breathe, and regulate body temperature; social pressures

2. Identify two causes of overweight. ____________________________
   (List 2:) heredity, medical problems, overeating (Students may also indicate specific social or emotional reasons people overeat.)

3. What five factors affect your daily calorie need? sex, age, size, body composition, and level of activity

4. Give two tips for successful weight loss. (Answers will vary.)

5. Explain the basics of planning a good weight management plan.____________________________
   A good weight management plan is part of a lifestyle that involves using food choices and exercise to reach and/or maintain a healthy weight.

Eating Disorders—Characteristics and Treatment

Activity E   Name _______________________________

Chapter 5   Date _______________________ Period ___________

Identify the eating disorder described by each of the following statements. Write *AN* in the blank if the statement describes anorexia nervosa. Write *BN* in the blank if the statement describes bulimia nervosa. Write *BED* in the blank if the statement describes binge eating disorder.

_AN_   1. A person with this disorder has a distorted body image, seeing himself or herself as fat regardless of actual appearance.

_AN_   2. This disorder causes blood pressure and body temperature to drop and respiration to slow.

_BN_   3. People with this disorder feel a lack of control over their eating behaviors.

BED   4. People with this disorder are often overweight.

_BN_   5. This disorder frequently damages the teeth, gums, esophagus, and stomach.

_AN_   6. A person with this disorder does not realize he or she has an eating disorder.

_BN_   7. People with this disorder may experience fatigue and heart abnormalities as results of a chemical imbalance due to frequent purging.

_AN_   8. This disorder is characterized by self-starvation.

BED   9. This disorder involves eating binges that are not followed by any effort to prevent weight gain.

_BN_   10. This disorder involves eating binges followed by a behavior to prevent weight gain.

Answer the following questions about treatment for eating disorders.

11. What type of treatment improves the chance of recovery from an eating disorder with no severe health problems?

    early treatment

12. Why might a person with an eating disorder require hospitalization? _______________________

    to treat symptoms of malnutrition or other damage to the body

13. Explain what role each of the following health professionals might play in the treatment of an eating disorder.

    A. physician Treat physical effects of the disorder.

    B. psychological counselor Provide individual, family, and group therapy to support the disordered eater.

    C. registered dietitian Help the patient learn how to make nutritious food choices.

    D. fitness counselor Set up a sound program of physical activity.

14. How can family members help a person with an eating disorder? _______________________

    Family members can learn to address issues that may have triggered the eating disorder. They can also offer support as the person with an eating disorder works to change his or her behavior.

15. How can a friend help someone he or she suspects has an eating disorder? _______________________

    Confront the person privately. Be honest. Express care and support. Suggest the person see a professional about behaviors that have caused concern.

   Guide to Good Food Workbook

Safeguarding Health

Health Beat

Activity A   Name _______________________________________

Chapter 6   Date _________________________   Period _____________

Presume you are a reporter for a local newspaper who writes a regular column called *Health Beat*. One of your contacts at the local hospital calls to tell you it looks like there has been an outbreak of foodborne illness. As you investigate, you take the notes shown below. Use the notes to write an eye-catching headline and an article about what happened. Be sure your article answers the questions jotted at the bottom of your notes. Write your article in the space provided.

15 people treated and released

1 person hospitalized — 78-year-old Agnes Simpson

All reported bloody stools, nausea, and vomiting

Symptoms appeared 12-15 hours after eating at Jake's Diner

All ate rare or medium hamburgers

- *What is the cause of these illnesses?*
- *Why was Mrs. Simpson hospitalized if all others were treated and released?*
- *How could this outbreak have been prevented?*

(Answers will vary.)

A Not-So-Safe Supper

Activity B   **Name** ___________________________________

Chapter 6   **Date** _________________________   **Period** ____________

Read the following story. In the space provided at the bottom of the page, list 10 guidelines for keeping food safe that Gina failed to follow. Identify which of the four basic steps to food safety—clean, separate, cook, and chill—each guideline represents.

Gina is a live-in cook at Siloam House, a group home for developmentally disabled adults. She'd spent the afternoon working in Siloam's vegetable garden with the activity therapist and some of the residents and had lost track of time. Now Gina was getting a late start preparing dinner. She rushed into the kitchen and set the just-picked tomatoes on the counter. Then she decided to get the meat loaf into the oven before going to her quarters to shower and change.

As Gina bent over to get a large bowl out of the cabinet, her long hair tumbled over her shoulders. She quickly brushed her hair aside with her hands and went about her work.

This morning, Gina left the ground beef on the kitchen counter to thaw. Now that it was defrosted, Gina unwrapped it and put it in the bowl. Then she got an onion out of a sack under the kitchen sink. As Gina started chopping the onion, some of the juice got into a cut on her finger and made her wince in pain.

Gina mixed the chopped onion and other ingredients with the ground beef in the bowl. Then she turned the mixture out onto a cutting board and shaped it into a loaf with her hands. Gina placed the meat loaf in a baking pan and put it in the oven.

Gina wiped her hands on a dishtowel. Then she began tearing lettuce into a bowl for a salad. Gina cut one of the tomatoes from the garden on the cutting board she'd used for the meat loaf. She arranged the tomato wedges on top of the lettuce.

As she put the salad in the refrigerator, Gina got out a raw egg, lemon juice, and Parmesan cheese. She combined these ingredients with olive oil to make her famous Caesar dressing.

Just then, Morris, Siloam's housecat, came into the kitchen. "I guess it's time for your dinner, too," Gina said. She opened a can of cat food and emptied it into a dish on the floor beside the refrigerator.

With only 30 minutes until dinnertime, Gina went to her quarters to take a shower. On returning to the kitchen after showering, Gina peered through the oven window. The meat loaf looked done, so she took it out of the oven and called the residents and staff to the dinner table.

(List 10 total:) *Clean*—Gina did not wash her hands before beginning work, Gina was not wearing clean clothes or a clean apron. Gina did not tie back her hair. Gina did not wash her hands after touching her hair. Gina stored her onions under the kitchen sink. Gina handled food when she had an open cut on her finger. Gina did not wash her hands or the cutting board after handling raw meat. Gina used a dishtowel to wipe her hands. Gina did not wash the lettuce or tomato before making the salad. *Separate*—Gina used the same cutting board for raw meat and fresh tomatoes. Gina fed the cat in the kitchen. *Cook*—Gina used uncooked egg in her salad dressing. Gina did not use a food thermometer to check the temperature of the meat loaf before removing it from the oven. *Chill*—Gina thawed the ground beef on the kitchen counter.

      Copyright by Goodheart-Willcox Co., Inc.

Temperature Control

Activity C   Name ____

Chapter 6   Date _____________________________   Period ____________

Choose the temperature that best answers each question. Write the letter in the space provided.

		°F
__H__	1. At what minimum temperature should hot foods be held?	
__G__	2. What is the recommended internal temperature for cooked cuts of meat, such as beef steaks and roasts?	A. 240
		B. 212
__F__	3. What is the recommended internal temperature for cooked ground beef?	C. 180
__E__	4. What is the recommended internal temperature for cooked whole poultry?	D. 170
		E. 165
__E__	5. What is the recommended internal temperature for cooked chicken breast pieces?	F. 160
		G. 145
__E__	6. What is the recommended temperature for reheating leftovers?	H. 140
__K__	7. At what maximum temperature should cold foods be held?	I. 126
__K, H__	8. What are the end points of the danger zone—the temperature range at which bacteria multiply fastest?	J. 60
		K. 40
__K__	9. What is the maximum temperature at which a refrigerator should be set?	L. 32
__M__	10. What is the maximum temperature at which a freezer should be set?	M. 0

Provide complete responses to the following questions. Write your responses in the space provided.

11. What is the maximum amount of time perishable foods can safely be held in the danger zone?

    two hours

12. How should low-acid, home-canned foods be prepared? ___________________

    They should be boiled for 10 to 20 minutes before tasting.

13. How should foods be packaged for the freezer? ___________________

    They should be wrapped in moistureproof and vaporproof wraps.

14. How can refrigerated foods be cooled faster? ___________________

    Use shallow storage containers and/or place containers of food in an ice-water bath.

15. How can foods served buffet style be kept at safe temperatures? Put food in small serving dishes, which can be refilled or replaced as needed. Use heated serving appliances and ice.

16. How can picnic and barbecue foods be kept at safe temperatures? Use insulated containers. Keep beverages in a separate cooler. Keep perishables in the cooler until you are ready to cook or serve them.

17. In terms of temperature, how should foods be served in a restaurant? ___________________

    Hot foods should be served hot. Cold foods should be served cold.

18. What food safety guideline should be followed regarding leftovers from a restaurant? ___________________

    If you cannot refrigerate food within two hours from the time it was served, discard it.

Handling Emergencies

Activity D   **Name** _______________________________________

Chapter 6   **Date** ____________________   **Period** ___________

Indicate the most appropriate response to each of the following emergency situations. Write your responses in the space provided.

1. You get a minor cut on your knuckle while grating cheese. What do you do?___________

   Apply pressure to stop any bleeding. Wash the cut with soap and water. Then apply an antiseptic solution and bandage the cut with a sterile dressing.

2. You burn the back of your hand on an oven rack. What do you do? _________________

   Immediately place the burned area under cold running water or in a cold-water bath.

3. Your coworker falls off a step stool, and you think his ankle may be broken. What do you do? ________

   Do not move your coworker or give him anything to eat or drink. Make him as comfortable as possible and call a physician.

4. A child in your care has just swallowed some type of cleaning fluid in an unlabeled bottle. What do you do?

   Call the poison control center and describe the product the child swallowed.

5. You find a prep cook lying on the kitchen floor. A portable mixer, still plugged in, is in the sink and the water is running. You suspect the worker has received an electric shock. What do you do?

   Immediately turn off the power and the water and then disconnect the mixer to avoid further danger of shock. Call your local emergency number.

6. You are having dinner with a client when she suddenly puts her hand to her throat. She cannot speak and her face is beginning to turn blue. What do you do?

   The client is choking. Perform the abdominal thrust.

7. You gash your wrist with a cleaver. Blood is spurting out of the deep wound. What do you do?

   Cover the wound with a sterile cloth or clean handkerchief. Apply firm pressure and have someone take you to a doctor or the hospital emergency room.

8. An older gentleman eats chicken for dinner. Later, he complains of a severe headache, abdominal pain, and vomiting. You suspect he is suffering from salmonellosis. What do you do?

   As an older adult, the gentleman is at greater risk from the salmonellosis infection. You should take him to a doctor.

   Guide to Good Food Workbook

Kitchen and Dining Areas

Kitchen Floor Plans

Activity A Name _______________________________

Chapter 7 Date _______________________ Period ___________

Complete the following exercises related to kitchen floor plans. Write your responses in the space provided.

(The three points of the triangle should be labeled: food preparation and storage center, cooking and serving center, cleanup center.)

1. Label the three major work centers of the work triangle to the left.

2. What should the maximum length of the three sides of the work triangle be? _21 feet (6.3 m)_

3. What additional work centers might be found in a kitchen? _________
   mixing center, planning center, laundry center, eating center
   ____

4. Label each of the kitchen floor plans that follow and draw in the work triangle.

A. _peninsula kitchen_

B. _U-shaped kitchen_

C. _corridor kitchen_

D. _L-shaped kitchen_

E. _one-wall kitchen_

F. _island kitchen_

5. Which plan is considered the most desirable? _U-shaped kitchen_
   Why? _because of its compact work triangle_

6. Which plan can easily include an eating area or another built-in appliance? _peninsula kitchen_

7. In which kitchen may traffic interfere with the work triangle? _corridor kitchen_

8. Which plan is most often found in apartments? _one-wall kitchen_
   Name a disadvantage of this plan. _lacks adequate storage or counters; long, narrow work triangle_

9. In which plan does a counter stand alone in the center of the room? _island kitchen_

10. Which plan can easily adapt to a variety of room arrangements? _L-shaped kitchen_

Kitchen Surface and Fixture Analysis

Activity B **Name** _______________________________________

Chapter 7 **Date** _______________________ **Period** ___________

Put yourself in the role of an interior designer who specializes in kitchen design. When addressing the surfaces and fixtures in a kitchen, asking a variety of questions allows you to determine how your clients feel about their present kitchen space. Answer the following questions about surfaces and fixtures in your home kitchen to help better relate to the needs and desires expressed by your clients. Write your responses in the space provided.

1. What wall covering material is used in your kitchen? (Answers will vary.) _______________

2. Do you like this material? Explain why or why not. (Answers will vary.) _______________

    ____

3. What do you consider to be the most important factor when choosing a kitchen wall covering?
    (Answers will vary.) ____

    ____

4. If you were re-covering your kitchen walls, what material would you choose? Explain your choice.
    (Answers will vary.) ____

    ____

5. What floor covering material is used in your kitchen? (Answers will vary.) _______________

6. Do you like this material? Explain why or why not. (Answers will vary.) _______________

    ____

7. What do you consider to be the most important factor when choosing a kitchen floor covering?
    (Answers will vary.) ____

    ____

8. If you were re-covering your kitchen floors, what material would you choose? Explain your choice.
    (Answers will vary.) ____

    ____

9. What countertop material is used in your kitchen? (Answers will vary.) _______________

10. Do you like this material? Explain why or why not. (Answers will vary.) _______________

    ____

11. What do you consider to be the most important factor when choosing a countertop material?
    (Answers will vary.) ____

    ____

12. If you were replacing your kitchen countertops, what material would you choose? Explain your choice.
    (Answers will vary.) ____

    ____

(Continued)

13. What cabinet material is used in your kitchen? (Answers will vary.) _______________________

14. Do you like this material? Explain why or why not. (Answers will vary.) _________________

____

____

15. What do you consider to be the most important factor when choosing kitchen cabinets?

    (Answers will vary.) ____

____

16. What, if anything, do you store in your kitchen cabinets other than food preparation and storage items?

    (Answers will vary.) ____

____

17. What, if any, special storage features do your cabinets offer? (Answers will vary.) _________

____

18. If you were replacing your kitchen cabinets, what material would you choose? Explain your choice.

    (Answers will vary.) ____

____

19. If you were replacing your kitchen cabinets, what additional special storage features would you choose? Explain your choice.

    (Answers will vary.) ____

____

20. What are the sources of natural light in your kitchen? (Answers will vary.) ________________

21. What are the sources of artificial lighting in your kitchen? Identify whether they provide general lighting or task lighting.

    (Answers will vary.) ____

____

22. What, if any, need do you have for additional lighting in your kitchen? (Answers will vary.) ___

____

23. What are the sources of ventilation in your kitchen? (Answers will vary.) _________________

____

24. What, if any, need do you have for additional ventilation? (Answers will vary.) ____________

____

25. How many electrical outlets do you have in your kitchen? (Answers will vary.) _____________

26. What, if any, need do you have for additional electrical outlets in your kitchen? (Answers will vary.)

____

____

Choosing Table Appointments

Activity C   Name ____

Chapter 7   Date ______________________________   Period ____________

Imagine you are a banquet manager at a large hotel. Your hotel has a wide variety of table appointments available to help set just the right mood at any type of event. However, in keeping with the hotel's environmentally friendly *green* policies, you do not offer disposable table appointments as an option. Check the appropriate blanks for the types of table appointments you would suggest to each of the clients described in the following. Then describe suggestions for centerpieces, colors, and designs in the space provided. Finally, use the space for notes to explain the reasons for each of your suggestions.

1. Cynthia VanCleef and her fiancé, Rodney Wellington, are planning a formal, adults-only evening wedding reception for 300 guests. This event will be held in the Grande Ballroom. Cynthia's wedding colors are pale pink and chocolate brown.   (Answers will vary.)

   Dinnerware: _____ china _____ stoneware/earthenware/pottery _____ glass-ceramic _____ plastic

   Flatware: _____ sterling silver _____ silver plate _____ stainless steel

   Beverageware: _____ lead glass _____ lime glass _____ plastic

   Holloware: _____ matching _____ complementary

   Table linens: _____ tablecloths _____ place mats _____ table runners

   Napkins: _____ matching _____ contrasting

   Centerpieces: (Answers will vary.) ____

   Colors/designs: (Answers will vary.) ____

   Notes: (Answers will vary.) ____

   ____

   ____

2. Vincent Howsier is hosting an afternoon Hawaiian luau for his sales staff and their families to reward them for exceeding the company's annual sales goals. Vincent is expecting about 125 people to attend the event, which will be held outdoors on the deck surrounding the Turquoise Pool.   (Answers will vary.)

   Dinnerware: _____ china _____ stoneware/earthenware/pottery _____ glass-ceramic _____ plastic

   Flatware: _____ sterling silver _____ silver plate _____ stainless steel

   Beverageware: _____ lead glass _____ lime glass _____ plastic

   Holloware: _____ matching _____ complementary

   Table linens: _____ tablecloths _____ place mats _____ table runners

   Napkins: _____ matching _____ contrasting

   Centerpieces: (Answers will vary.) ____

   Colors/designs: (Answers will vary.) ____

   Notes: (Answers will vary.) ____

   ____

   ____

(Continued)

3. Abby Clayton is holding a brainstorming brunch for the agents of the Gold Star Real Estate Agency. She has invited about 25 agents from three offices in the metropolitan area. She wants the event to be casual but businesslike. It will be held in Conference Room A.   (Answers will vary.)

   Dinnerware: _____ china   _____ stoneware/earthenware/pottery   _____ glass-ceramic   _____ plastic

   Flatware: _____ sterling silver   _____ silver plate   _____ stainless steel

   Beverageware: _____ lead glass   _____ lime glass   _____ plastic

   Holloware: _____ matching   _____ complementary

   Table linens: _____ tablecloths   _____ place mats   _____ table runners

   Napkins: _____ matching   _____ contrasting

   Centerpieces: (Answers will vary.) ____

   Colors/designs: (Answers will vary.) ____

   Notes: (Answers will vary.) ____

   ____

   ____

4. Carter Blackwell is the campaign manager for Diane Habbingdon, who is running for state treasurer. Carter is planning a meet-and-greet reception for about 100 potential campaign contributors. Carter wants several appetizer and drink stations placed throughout the room. Although there will be a couple groupings of chairs for those who want to sit and converse, most of the guests will stand and eat as they mingle. The event is scheduled from 4:00 to 7:00 PM in the Jefferson Meeting Room.   (Answers will vary.)

   Dinnerware: _____ china   _____ stoneware/earthenware/pottery   _____ glass-ceramic   _____ plastic

   Flatware: _____ sterling silver   _____ silver plate   _____ stainless steel

   Beverageware: _____ lead glass   _____ lime glass   _____ plastic

   Holloware: _____ matching   _____ complementary

   Table linens: _____ tablecloths   _____ place mats   _____ table runners

   Napkins: _____ matching   _____ contrasting

   Centerpieces: (Answers will vary.) ____

   Colors/designs: (Answers will vary.) ____

   Notes: (Answers will vary.) ____

   ____

   ____

Setting the Table

Name ________________________________

Date ________________________ Period ____________

Using the rectangles below as place mats, draw an individual cover for each of the following menus. Each cover should include the correct placement of the dinnerware, flatware, beverageware, and linens needed by one person. Label or draw the menu items for each cover as shown in the following example.

Steak
Baked Potato
Tossed Salad
Texas Toast
Strawberry Ice Cream
Iced Tea

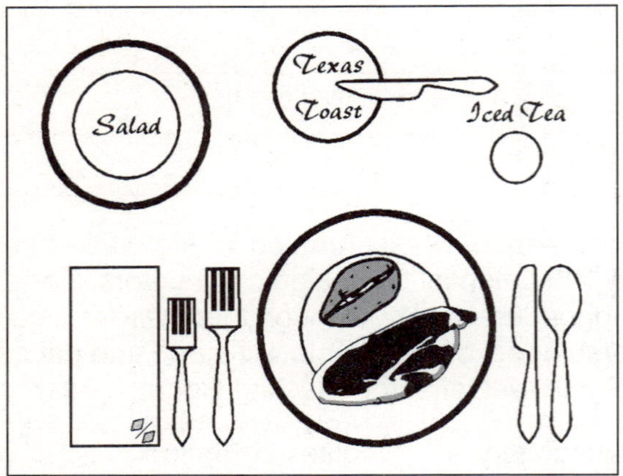

(Ice cream is served when dinner is removed.)

Orange Juice
Oatmeal
Muffin
Milk

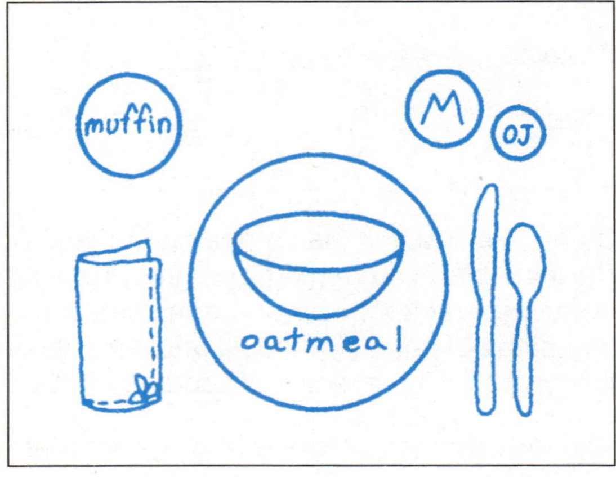

Tuna Sandwich
Celery and Carrot Sticks
Cookies
Milk

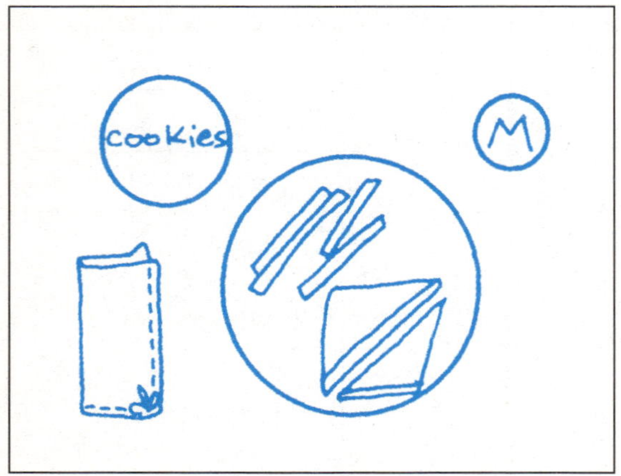

Barbecued Chicken
Mashed Potatoes
Broccoli
Dinner Rolls
Apple Pie
Milk

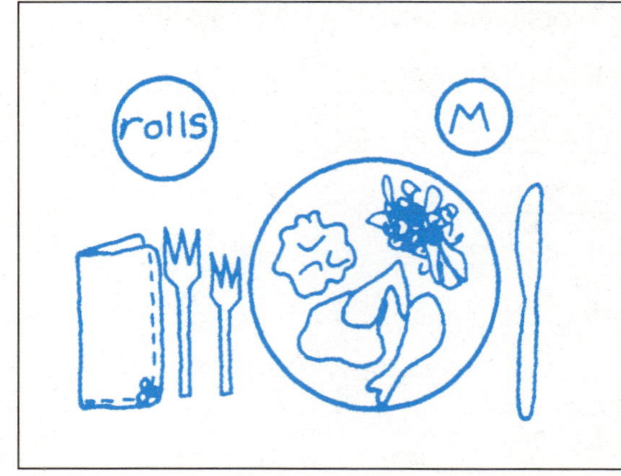

(Pie served when dinner is removed.)

Kitchen Appliances

Comparing Energy Labeling

Activity A   Name ____

Chapter 8   Date ____________________________   Period ____________

Use the EnergyGuide labels to answer the questions that follow. Write your responses in the space provided.

Model A

Model B

1. What type and style of appliance do these labels describe? _top-mount refrigerator_

2. Which model has the larger capacity? _Model A_

3. Which model has the lower estimated yearly operating cost? _Model A_

4. What is the difference in estimated yearly operating cost between the two models? _$7.00_

5. What is the estimated yearly electricity use of Model B? _479 kWh_

6. Why might a consumer's actual operating cost differ from the estimate shown on the label?
   The cost will depend on utility rates and use.

7. How can consumers tell which model is better for the environment? ______________________
   Model A is better for the environment because it has earned the ENERGY STAR rating.

8. Suppose Model A costs $799 and Model B costs $649. You expect to own this appliance for 12 years. Which model would you choose? Explain your answer on a separate sheet of paper. _(Answers will vary.)_

Selecting Major Appliances

Name ____

Date ______________________________   Period ____________

Imagine you are a property manager hired by an investment group. The group has purchased several new condominium units, which will soon be advertised as vacation rental properties in a resort community. The group has chosen units with various floor plans to appeal to a range of guests. One of your responsibilities is to choose the major kitchen appliances best suited to each unit. Read the following descriptions and then answer the questions about the appliances you will choose.

1. Large four-bedroom, two-bath ocean-view units are likely to be rented by two or three families who are vacationing together. From your experience, you know these families often enjoy doing some gourmet cooking during their vacation stays. Place a check mark to the left of the cooking appliances you will choose for these units. (Answers will vary.)

   A. What type of fuel will the cooking appliances use?
   _____ electric   _____ gas   _____ dual-fuel

   B. What style of cooking appliances will you choose?
   _____ separate built-in cooktop and oven   _____ freestanding range   _____ slide-in/drop-in range

   C. What oven arrangement will you choose?
   _____ single conventional oven   _____ single combination oven with convection cooking
   _____ double oven: one conventional, one convection

   D. Explain your cooking appliance choices. (Answers will vary.) __________________

   ____

   ____

   E. What care instructions for the cooking appliances will you give to the daily housekeeping staff?

   (Answers will vary.) ____

   ____

2. One-room efficiency suites are likely to be rented by business travelers looking for more space and affordability than offered by local hotels. After long days of business meetings, these guests often bring in takeout food or prepare frozen entrees picked up from a nearby convenience store. Place a check mark to the left of the type of microwave oven you will choose for the fully-equipped mini kitchens in these units. (Answers will vary.)

   A. What is the primary type of cooking for which the microwave oven will be used?
   _____ full cooking   _____ defrosting   _____ reheating

   B. How many power levels should the microwave have?
   _____ multiple power levels   _____ single power level

   C. What style of microwave oven will you choose?
   _____ countertop   _____ combination microwave and hood

   D. Explain your microwave oven choices. (Answers will vary.) __________________

   ____

   ____

   E. What care instructions for the microwave oven will you give to the daily housekeeping staff?

   (Answers will vary.) ____

   ____

(Continued)

3. Cozy one-bedroom units with fireplaces and whirlpool tubs are most likely to appeal to couples enjoying romantic getaways. The couples will likely eat many of their meals in some of the area's best-known restaurants. The kitchens in the one-bedroom units are equipped with more basic appliances than the larger units. Place a check mark to the left of the type of refrigerator you will choose for the kitchens in these units. (Answers will vary.)

   A. What capacity refrigerator will you choose?
   _____ less than 15 cubic feet   _____ 15.1 to 19 cubic feet   _____ 19.1 to 23 cubic feet
   _____ 23.1 to 26 cubic feet

   B. What style of refrigerator will you choose?
   _____ top-mount   _____ side-by-side   _____ bottom-mount

   C. What type of frost management will you choose?
   _____ frost free   _____ manual defrost

   D. Explain your refrigerator choices. (Answers will vary.) ___________________________

   ____

   ____

   E. What care instructions for the refrigerator will you give to the daily housekeeping staff?

   (Answers will vary.) ____

   ____

4. Two-bedroom units will probably most often be rented by single families. You expect these families to prepare many of their meals in the unit to save the costs of eating out. However, they are likely to focus on quick, simple foods so they have more time to spend enjoying the beach and other local attractions. Place a check mark to the left of the type of dishwasher you will choose for the kitchens in the two-bedroom units. (Answers will vary.)

   A. Do you want a dishwasher that has earned the ENERGY STAR?
   _____ yes   _____ no   _____ maybe

   B. What wash cycles do you want the dishwasher to offer? (Check all that apply.)
   _____ speed cycle   _____ sanitizing   _____ heavy duty/pots and pans   _____ delayed wash

   C. What style of dishwasher will you choose?
   _____ built-in   _____ portable

   D. Explain your dishwasher choices. (Answers will vary.) ___________________________

   ____

   ____

   E. What care instructions for the dishwasher will you give to the daily housekeeping staff?

   (Answers will vary.) ____

   ____

Portable Appliance Performance Comparison

Activity C   **Name** ____

Chapter 8   **Date** ___________________________   **Period** ____________

Choose two portable appliances that perform the same basic tasks. (Possible choices include standard mixer and hand mixer, blender and food processor, toaster and toaster-oven, and electric percolator and automatic drip coffeemaker.) Prepare the same simple food product with both appliances. Then complete the comparison that follows.

1. Food product prepared: (Answers will vary.) _______________________________

2. Preparation step(s) completed by the appliances: (Answers will vary.) _______________

3. (Chart answers will vary.)

Appliance A	Appliance B
________________________	________________________
Convenience features	Convenience features
Safety features	Safety features
Advantages	Advantages
Disadvantages	Disadvantages

4. Which appliance do you feel did a better job of preparing the food product? (Answers will vary.) _______

   Why? (Answers will vary.) ____

5. For what types of food products might the other appliance be preferred? (Answers will vary.) _______

   Why? (Answers will vary.) ____

6. Which appliance is easier to operate? (Answers will vary.) _______________________

   Why? (Answers will vary.) ____

7. Which appliance is easier to clean? (Answers will vary.) _______________________

   Why? (Answers will vary.) ____

8. Which appliance would be easier to store? (Answers will vary.) ___________________

   Why? (Answers will vary.) ____

9. Which appliance would you rather own? (Answers will vary.) ____________________

   Why? (Answers will vary.) ____

10. Do you think it would be worthwhile to own both appliances? (Answers will vary.) _______

    Why or why not? (Answers will vary.) ______________________________________

Kitchen Utensils

Small Equipment Identification

Activity A   **Name** ____

Chapter 9   **Date** ____________________________   **Period** ____________

Identify the following equipment names and types (measuring tool, mixing tool, baking tool, thermometer, cutting tool, or other preparation tool) and describe the uses of each. Write your responses in the space provided.

1. Name: _measuring spoons_

   Type: _measuring tool_

   Uses: _(Answers will vary.)_

2. Name: _flexible spatula_

   Type: _baking tool_

   Uses: _(Answers will vary.)_

3. Name: _tongs_

   Type: _other preparation tool_

   Uses: _(Answers will vary.)_

4. Name: _peeler_

   Type: _cutting tool_

   Uses: _(Answers will vary.)_

5. Name: _straight-edged spatula_

   Type: _baking tool_

   Uses: _(Answers will vary.)_

(Continued)

6.

Name: slotted spoon

Type: mixing tool

Uses: (Answers will vary.)

____

7.

Name: liquid measures

Type: measuring tool

Uses: (Answers will vary.)

____

8.

Name: whisk

Type: mixing tool

Uses: (Answers will vary.)

____

9.

Name: chef's knife (French)

Type: cutting tool

Uses: (Answers will vary.)

____

10.

Name: sifter

Type: baking tool

Uses: (Answers will vary.)

____

11.

Name: rolling pin

Type: baking tool

Uses: (Answers will vary.)

____

12.

Name: kitchen shears

Type: cutting tool

Uses: (Answers will vary.)

____

13.

Name: shredder-grater

Type: cutting tool

Uses: (Answers will vary.)

____

(Continued)

14. Name: baster
Type: other preparation tool
Uses: (Answers will vary.)

15. Name: strainer
Type: other preparation tool
Uses: (Answers will vary.)

16. Name: pastry blender
Type: baking tool
Uses: (Answers will vary.)

17. Name: rotary beater
Type: mixing tool
Uses: (Answers will vary.)

18. Name: ladle
Type: other preparation tool
Uses: (Answers will vary.)

19. 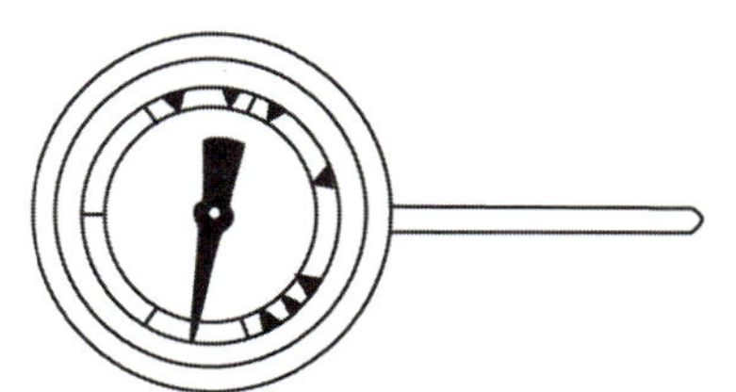
Name: dry measures
Type: measuring tool
Uses: (Answers will vary.)

20 Name: meat thermometer
Type: thermometer
Uses: (Answers will vary.)

Materials Comparison

Name _______________________________

Date ___________________________ Period ___________

Complete the following chart by giving the advantages and disadvantages of each of the cookware and bakeware materials listed. Then answer the questions that follow. Write your responses in the space provided. (Chart answers will vary.)

Material	Advantages	Disadvantages
Cast iron		
Aluminum		
Copper		
Stainless steel		
Glass		
Glass-ceramic		
Porcelain enamel		
Ceramic materials		
Silicone and Plastic		

1. Which material would be your first choice for rangetop cookware? (Answers will vary.) _____________

   Why? (Answers will vary.) ____

   ____

2. Which material would be your first choice for conventional bakeware? (Answers will vary.) _________

   Why? (Answers will vary.) ____

   ____

3. Which material would be your first choice for microwave bakeware? (Answers will vary.) __________

   Why? (Answers will vary.) ____

   ____

Microwave Cookware

Explain why each of the following statements about microwave cookware is false. Write your responses in the space provided.

1. Microwaves should be reflected by microwave cookware. ____________________________

   Microwaves should be able to pass through microwave cookware to allow them to reach the food.

   ____

2. Microwaves can pass through metal. ____________________________

   Microwaves can pass through materials such as ceramic, plastics, glass, wood, and paper. Metal cookware reflects microwaves.

3. Metal should never be used in a microwave oven. ____________________________

   Although metal cookware is generally not recommended for microwave use, some browning dishes with metal cooking surfaces are specially designed for microwave use.

4. A platter with silver or gold trim would be attractive for both cooking and serving foods prepared in a microwave oven.

   Cookware made of microwavable material with bands of metal trim should not be used in the microwave oven because it can cause arcing.

5. Disposable plastic containers from margarine and whipped toppings are recommended for microwave cooking.

   Do not use disposable plastic containers from margarine or whipped toppings in the microwave. They are made of soft plastics that may melt from contact with hot food.

6. Wooden bowls are a good choice for microwaving liquids. ____________________________

   You should not use containers that absorb liquid, such as wooden bowls, when microwaving liquids. The moisture absorbed by such a container will attract microwave energy away from the food.

7. Square cookware pieces are the best shape for microwave cooking. ____________________________

   Round-shaped containers allow microwaves to hit food evenly. Microwaves can overlap in the corners of square cookware pieces, causing food in the corners to overcook.

8. Ring-shaped pans slow cooking time in a microwave oven. ____________________________

   Ring shapes allow microwaves to hit food from the center as well as the top, bottom, and sides, which speeds cooking time.

9. Always choose large cookware pieces to allow plenty of room for microwaves to circulate around food.

   Cookware pieces should correspond to the amount of food being microwaved.

10. A shallow container is a good choice for microwaving milk. ____________________________

    Milk can boil over in a shallow container.

Equipment Review

Name ___________________________________

Date _______________________ Period ____________

Each clue below describes a different piece of kitchen equipment. Using these clues, identify the piece of equipment described. Write your responses in the space provided.

whisk	1. I am preferred by most chefs for incorporating air into foods like soufflés and for preventing lumps from forming in sauces.
stockinette	2. I keep dough from sticking to a rolling pin.
pastry brush	3. I am used to brush butter or sauces on foods.
pastry blender	4. I am several thin, curved pieces of metal attached to a handle, and I am used for making pastry.
oven-safe thermometer	5. I am designed to be placed in food while it is cooking to register the internal temperature.
shredder-grater	6. I am a four-sided metal tool used to shred and grate foods such as cabbage and cheese.
kitchen shears	7. I have a variety of uses including snipping herbs; trimming vegetables; and cutting meat, dough, and pizza.
flexible spatula	8. I am used for scraping bowls and saucepans and for folding one ingredient into another.
peeler	9. I am used to remove the outer surface of fruits and vegetables.
liquid measures	10. I am made of glass or plastic, and I am used for measuring ingredients such as milk and vegetable oil.
dry measures	11. I am made of metal or plastic, and I am used for measuring ingredients such as flour and sugar.
measuring spoons	12. I am used to measure small amounts of liquid and dry ingredients.
rotary beater	13. I am used to beat, blend, and incorporate air into foods when my crank is turned.
rolling pin	14. I am used to roll dough or pastry.
colander	15. I am used to drain fruits, vegetables, and pasta.
chef's (French) knife	16. I am a versatile tool with a long, smooth blade for chopping, dicing, and mincing.
cutting board	17. I am used to protect countertops when chopping foods.
strainer	18. I am used to separate liquid and solid foods.
sifter	19. I am used to blend dry ingredients and remove lumps from powdered sugar.
double boiler	20. I consist of a small pan that fits into a larger pan, and I am used to cook foods gently.
skillet	21. I am used for panbroiling foods or for cooking foods in a small amount of fat.
griddle	22. I am a skillet without sides, and I am used for grilling sandwiches and making pancakes.
cookie sheet	23. I am a flat sheet made of metal, and I am used for baking cookies.
muffin pan	24. I am an oblong pan with round depressions.
baster	25. I use suction to collect juices from meat and poultry.

CHAPTER 10
Planning Meals

Planning for Nutrition

Activity A   **Name** ____

Chapter 10   **Date** ________________________   **Period** ____________

Complete the following statements about planning nutritious meals by using the terms below to fill in the blanks.

breakfast	dinner	meal pattern	protein
complex carbohydrates	fruit group	protein foods group	registered dietitian
course	lunch	menu	snacks
dessert	meal manager	MyPlate	whole grains

1. The person responsible for seeing that meals provide good nutrition to meet the needs of each person eating the meal is the _meal manager_.

2. An outline of the basic foods normally served at a meal, which is called a(n) _meal pattern_, can help meal managers plan.

3. A meal pattern based on _MyPlate_ can provide all the nutrients needed each day at any calorie level.

4. Eating _breakfast_ helps prevent a midmorning slump.

5. A good breakfast should be rich in sources of _complex carbohydrates_, such as toast and cereals, for energy.

6. Many meal managers use leftovers to prepare nutritious salads, casseroles, and sandwiches for _lunch_.

7. Serving a new dish, serving common foods in new ways, and varying preparation methods are ways to add variety to _dinner_.

8. Meal managers can offer fruits and vegetables, low-fat cheese, and nuts for _snacks_ that satisfy nutritional needs as well as hunger.

9. A(n) _menu_ listing the foods to be served at a meal can help meal managers assess whether they are serving foods from all the groups in MyPlate.

10. A part of a meal made up of all the foods served at one time is a(n) _course_.

11. Meal managers usually center their menus on a _protein_ food.

12. Begin meal planning by choosing a main dish, remembering that it does not have to be from the _protein foods group_.

13. Meal managers need to make sure at least half the grain foods chosen to accompany the main dish are _whole grains_.

14. Keeping calories in mind, meal managers can select a _dessert_ and/or first course, remembering to make nutrient-dense choices.

15. When planning for a family member with special needs, a meal manager can work with a(n) _registered dietitian_.

Planned Spending

Activity B Name _______________________________

Chapter 10 Date _____________________ Period ___________

Read the following statements about planned spending. Circle *T* if the statement is true or *F* if the statement is false.

T (F) 1. On the average, families in the United States spend about 50 percent of their income for food.

(T) F 2. It costs more to feed a teenager than it does to feed a senior citizen.

T (F) 3. All households with similar food needs spend the same amount of money on food.

T (F) 4. As income increases, the use of staple foods, such as beans and rice, tends to increase.

(T) F 5. Being able to recognize seasonal food values and choose quality meats and produce are important meal management skills.

(T) F 6. A meal manager's available time and energy affect the food budget.

T (F) 7. People who eat casseroles and canned goods will likely spend more on food than those who eat steaks and fresh produce.

T (F) 8. Value systems do not affect spending.

(T) F 9. A budget is a plan for managing income and expenses.

(T) F 10. A meal manager is responsible for staying within the budget when buying food.

(T) F 11. Money received as tips, gifts, and interest should usually not be included as sources of income in a budget.

T (F) 12. Savings should be listed on a budget as a flexible expense.

T (F) 13. Food and utility bills are examples of fixed expenses.

(T) F 14. Flexible expenses are easier to adjust than fixed expenses.

(T) F 15. Protein foods are the most costly group of foods.

(T) F 16. During off-seasons, canned and frozen fruits and vegetables are usually cheaper than fresh produce.

T (F) 17. Small packages of food products are usually better buys than large packages.

(T) F 18. A meal manager may be able to save money by preparing more foods from scratch.

(T) F 19. Restaurants, concession stands, and vending machines take a portion of food dollars.

(T) F 20. Overspending the food budget to stock up on sale items one week may enable a meal manager to underspend the next week.

Planning Satisfying Menus

Activity C　　　　**Name** _______________________________

Chapter 10　　　　**Date** ___________________________　　**Period** _____________

In the box below, create an illustration of a satisfying meal by either drawing various foods or clipping pictures from a magazine and mounting them. Then evaluate the meal by describing the variety it includes for each of the listed aspects of appetite appeal. Write your menu in the space provided following the illustration.

variety of colors _(Answers will vary.)_________________________________

variety of sizes _(Answers will vary.)_________________________________

variety of shapes _(Answers will vary.)_________________________________

variety of flavors _(Answers will vary.)_________________________________

variety of textures _(Answers will vary.)_________________________________

variety of temperatures _(Answers will vary.)_________________________________

(Illustrations will vary.)

Menu

____

____

____

____

____

Convenience Comparison

Activity D   **Name** ____

Chapter 10   **Date** _____________________________ **Period** _____________

Choose a food that is available in both semiprepared and finished convenience forms. Find a recipe for making this food and attach it to this page. Prepare the two convenience forms and the homemade form of this food and complete the chart that follows. Then answer the questions below the chart.

<table>
<tr><td colspan="2">Semiprepared</td><td colspan="2">Homemade</td></tr>
<tr><td>Ingredients</td><td>Cost</td><td>Ingredients</td><td>Cost</td></tr>
<tr><td>__________________</td><td>$ ________</td><td>__________________</td><td>$ ________</td></tr>
<tr><td>__________________</td><td>________</td><td>__________________</td><td>________</td></tr>
<tr><td>__________________</td><td>________</td><td>__________________</td><td>________</td></tr>
<tr><td>__________________</td><td>+ ________</td><td>__________________</td><td>________</td></tr>
<tr><td>Product cost</td><td>$ ________</td><td>__________________</td><td>________</td></tr>
<tr><td>Preparation time (in minutes)</td><td>________</td><td>__________________</td><td>________</td></tr>
<tr><td>Minimum wage per minute</td><td>× ___.12___</td><td>__________________</td><td>________</td></tr>
<tr><td>Labor cost</td><td>+ ________</td><td>__________________</td><td>+ ________</td></tr>
<tr><td>Total cost</td><td>$ ________</td><td>Product cost</td><td>$ ________</td></tr>
<tr><td colspan="2">Finished</td><td>Preparation time (in minutes)</td><td>________</td></tr>
<tr><td>Product cost</td><td>$ ________</td><td>Minimum wage per minute</td><td>× ___.12___</td></tr>
<tr><td>Preparation time (in minutes)</td><td>________</td><td>Labor cost</td><td>+ ________</td></tr>
<tr><td>Minimum wage per minute</td><td>× ___.12___</td><td>Total cost</td><td>$ ________</td></tr>
<tr><td>Labor cost</td><td>+ ________</td><td></td><td></td></tr>
<tr><td>Total cost</td><td>$ ________</td><td></td><td></td></tr>
</table>

	Total cost	÷	No. of servings	=	Cost per serving
A. Semiprepared	__________	÷	__________	=	__________
B. Finished	__________	÷	__________	=	__________
C. Homemade	__________	÷	__________	=	__________

1. How do the preparation times for the three products compare? _(Answers will vary.)_________

2. How does the cost per serving for each of the three products compare? _(Answers will vary.)_____

3. How do the appearance and flavor of the convenience products compare with those of the homemade product? _(Answers will vary.)____

4. Which product would you prefer to eat? _(Answers will vary.)_________________________

 Why? _(Answers will vary.)____

5. Which product would you prefer to make? _(Answers will vary.)_______________________

 Why? _(Answers will vary.)____

6. When might you use the other forms of this food? _(Answers will vary.)_________________

Shopping Decisions

Types of Stores

Activity A Name ________________________________

Chapter 11 Date ____________________________ Period ____________

Complete the following chart by describing the different types of food stores and listing the advantages and disadvantages of each. Then answer the questions that follow the chart. (Chart answers will vary.)

Type of Store	Description	Advantages	Disadvantages
Supermarket			
Discount supermarket			
Wholesale club			
Convenience store			
Specialty store			
Delicatessen			
Outlet store			
Food co-op			
Farmers' market			
Roadside stand			
Internet grocery store			

In which type of store would you prefer to shop? (Answers will vary.) ________________

Why? (Answers will vary.) ________________________________

When might you choose to shop for food in other types of stores? (Answers will vary.) ________

____

Using Food Advertisements

Activity B   **Name** _______________________________________

Chapter 11   **Date** ___________________________   **Period** ____________

Use the advertising flyer from a local supermarket to make a shopping list. Use the guide on the left to list the various specials according to the area of the store where you will find them. Then plan nutritious meals around the advertised specials in the spaces provided on the right. Write your responses in the space provided.

Shopping List

Produce

(Chart answers will vary.)

____

____

Dairy

____

____

____

Deli

____

____

____

Meat

____

____

Canned/packaged foods

____

____

Bakery

____

____

Frozen foods

____

____

Miscellaneous

____

____

____

Breakfast

(Answers will vary.)

____

____

____

____

____

Lunch

(Answers will vary.)

____

____

____

____

____

Dinner

(Answers will vary.)

____

____

____

____

____

Snacks

(Answers will vary.)

____

____

____

____

Unit Pricing

Compare the following pairs of shelf tags showing unit prices and answer the questions that follow in the space provided.

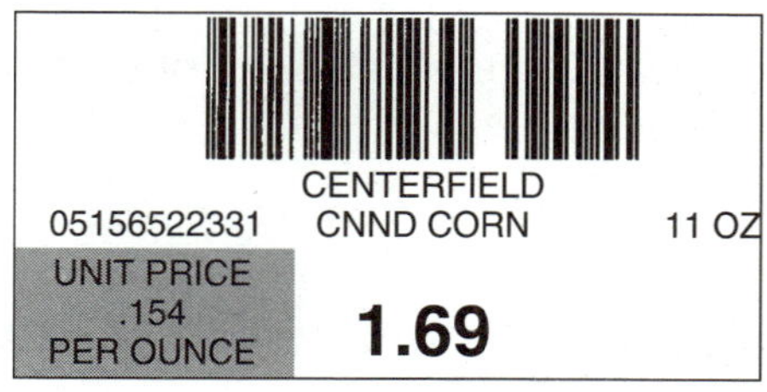

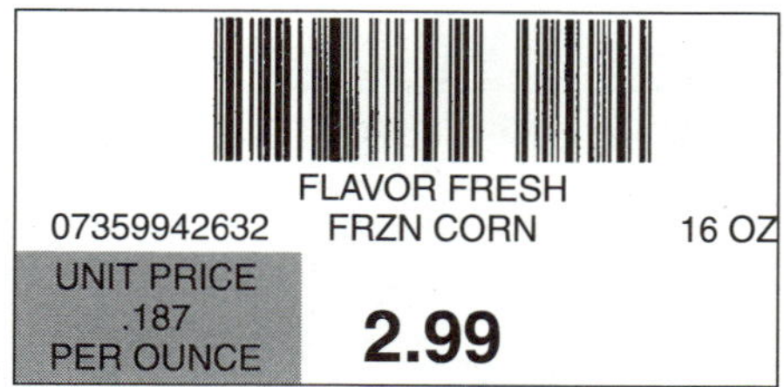

1. What is the total price of the canned corn? $1.69

2. What is the package size of the frozen corn? 16 ounces

3. Which form of corn has the lower unit price? canned

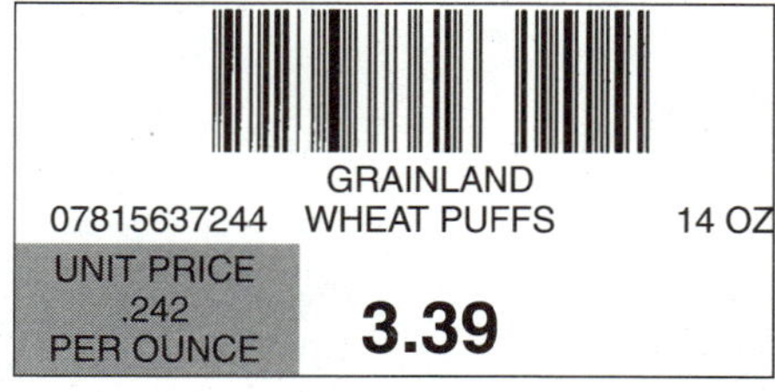

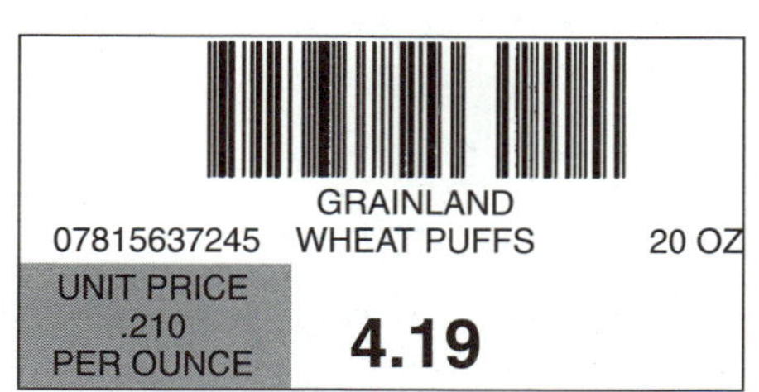

4. What size package of wheat puffs has the higher unit price? 14 ounces

5. What is the unit price of the 20-ounce package? .210 per ounce

6. What is the unit price difference between the two package sizes? .032 per ounce

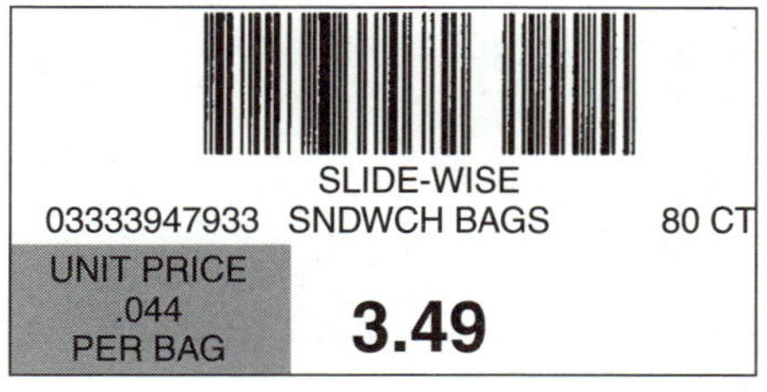

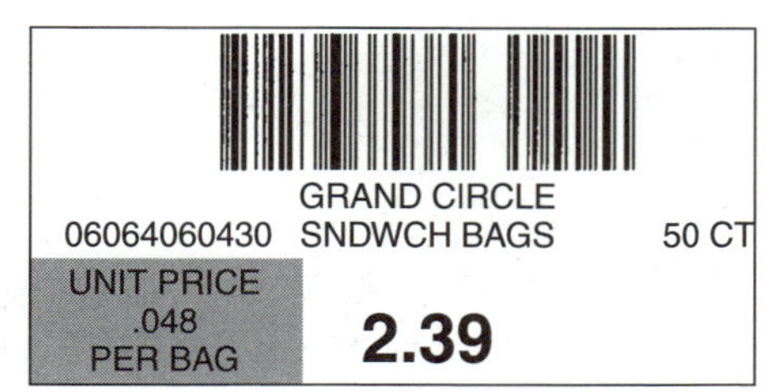

7. Which brand of sandwich bags has the lower total price? Grand Circle

8. Which brand has the lower unit price? Slide-Wise

9. How many bags are in a package of Grand Circle brand sandwich bags? 50

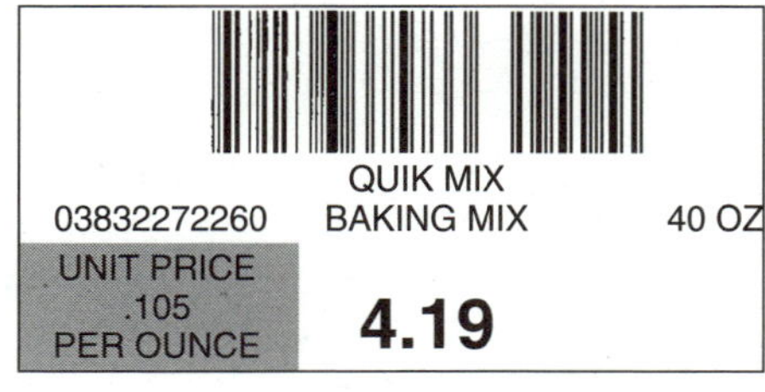

10. What type of product do these tags describe? baking mix

11. What is the unit price of the Quik Mix brand product? .105 per ounce

12. What brand comes in the smaller package? Grandma B's

Shopping Terminology

Name ___________________________

Date ___________________________   Period ___________

Complete the following statements about concepts that will help consumers make wise shopping decisions. Then arrange the circled letters to spell a shopping term. Answer the question that follows.

1. <u>Comparison shopping</u> involves evaluating different brands, sizes, and forms of a product before making a purchase decision.

2. A listing of a product's cost per standard unit, weight, or measure that generally appears on a shelf tag underneath the product is called <u>unit pricing</u>.

3. Many food products are given an indication of quality called a <u>grade</u>.

4. The name a manufacturer puts on products so people will know that company makes the products is called a <u>brand name</u>.

5. A brand sold only by a store or chain of stores is called a <u>store brand</u>.

6. Thinking about how packaging materials can be reused or recycled before buying a product is known as <u>precycling</u>.

7. <u>Organic foods</u> are foods produced without the use of synthetic fertilizers, pesticides, or growth stimulants.

8. Agents used to kill insects, weeds, and fungi that attack crops are called <u>pesticides</u>.

9. A substance that is added to food for a specific purpose, such as adding nutrients or preserving quality is called a <u>food additive</u>.

10. A food additive that sweetens foods without providing the calories of sugar is known as a(n) <u>artificial sweetener</u>.

11. A breakdown of how a food product fits in an average diet that appears on almost all food packages is <u>nutrition labeling</u>.

12. A series of lines, bars, and numbers that appears on packages of food and nonfood items to identify products is the <u>universal product code</u>.

13. <u>Open dating</u> uses calendar dates on perishable and semiperishable foods to help retailers know how long to display products.

Circled letters: <u>p, u, e, m, b, y, g, s, i, l, u, i, n</u>

Some people might say the opposite of comparison shopping is <u>impulse buying</u>.

14. What are three tips to help consumers avoid this practice when making shopping decisions?

(Answers will vary.)

____

____

____

Using Food Labeling

Activity E Name _______________________________________

Chapter 11 Date _______________________________ Period ____________

Use information on the package label shown to answer the following questions.

Grassy Meadow Farms

GRADE A
PASTEURIZED
HOMOGENIZED

FAT-FREE MILK VITAMIN A&D

Nutrition Facts

Serving Size 1 cup (240 mL)

Servings per container | About 8

Amount Per Serving

Calories 90	Calories from Fat 0

% Daily Value*

Total Fat 0g	0%
Saturated Fat 0g	0%
Trans Fat 0g	
Cholesterol Less than 5mg	1%
Sodium 120 mg	5%
Total Carbohydrate 13g	4%
Dietary Fiber 0g	0%
Sugars 13g	
Protein 9g	

Vitamin A 10%	*	Vitamin C 4%	
Calcium 30%	* Iron 0%	*	Vitamin D 25%

*Percent Daily Values are based on a 2,000 calorie diet. Your daily values may be higher or lower depending on your calorie needs:

	Calories:	2000	2,500
Total Fat	Less than	65g	80g
Sat Fat	Less than	20g	25g
Cholesterol	Less than	300mg	300mg
Sodium	Less than	2,400mg	2,400mg
Total Carbohydrate		300g	375g
Dietary Fiber		25g	30g

INGREDIENTS: FAT-FREE MILK, NONFAT DRY MILK, VITAMIN A PALMITATE, VITAMIN D_3.

0 37128 01016 3

KEEP REFRIGERATED
DIST BY
GRASSY MEADOW FARMS CO
FRANKLIN PARK IL 60131

SELL BY:	APR 09
MFG PLT:	1632
½ gal (1.89 L)	

1. What is the common name and form of this food?
   fat-free milk

2. What is the volume of the contents of this container?
   ½ gallon (1.89 L)

3. Who distributes this product? Grassy Meadow Farms Co.

4. What is the second most common ingredient in this product? nonfat dry milk

5. What is the size of a serving of this product? 1 cup

6. How many servings are in this container? about 8

7. How many calories does a serving of this product provide? 90 calories

8. How many grams of total fat does a serving of this product provide? 0 grams

9. What percent of the Daily Value for saturated fat does a serving of this product provide? 0 percent

10. What is the unit used to measure cholesterol in food products? milligrams (mg)

11. Would this product be considered high or low in sodium? low

12. How much of the carbohydrate in a serving of this product comes from sugars? all of it (13 g)

13. Is this product a better source of vitamin A or vitamin C? Explain your answer.
    It is a better source of vitamin A, providing 10 percent of the Daily Value. It provides only 4 percent of vitamin C.

14. How many servings of this product would a person need to receive 100 percent of the Daily Value for calcium? 3⅓ servings

15. How much fiber does a person on a 2,500-calorie diet need each day? 30 grams

16. Which nutrients does a serving of this product provide in high amounts? calcium, vitamin D

17. What is the UPC number of this product? 037128010163

18. How much protein does a serving of this product provide? 9 grams

19. What type of date appears on this product? sell-by date

20. What does this date tell you?
    It is the last day a store should sell the product.

Consumer Resources

Name _______________________________

Date _______________________ Period ___________

Identify which source of consumer help and information you would rely on in each of the following situations and your reason for choosing each source. Write your responses in the space provided.

1. You want to be sure there is not an unsafe amount of pesticide residue on the fruit you are buying.

   (Answers will vary.)

2. You want to be sure the meat you are buying has met standards for safety and wholesomeness.

   (Answers will vary.)

3. You buy a carton of milk from the store and find it is sour.

   (Answers will vary.)

4. After several complaints to the supermarket manager, you are still noticing prices ringing up at the register that do not match shelf tag prices.

   (Answers will vary.)

5. At the Cozy Cup Coffee Shop, the cream curdles when you pour it into your coffee and your scrambled eggs are undercooked. You also observe a server clearing dirty tables and then serving a food order without washing her hands.

   (Answers will vary.)

6. You open a can of chicken noodle soup. You find the can full of broth, vegetables, and noodles, but you cannot find one piece of chicken.

   (Answers will vary.)

7. When you open a box of cereal, you see the free toy inside has broken into small pieces, which are scattered throughout the box.

   (Answers will vary.)

8. You hear on the evening news about a recall of Kitchen Kettle chili. You want to find out if the two cans of chili on your pantry shelf are included in the recall.

   (Answers will vary.)

Recipes and Work Plans

Reading a Recipe

Activity A   **Name** ____________________________________

Chapter 12   **Date** ____________________________ **Period** ____________

Use the recipe below to answer the questions that follow. Write your responses in the space provided.

Vegetable Pasta Soup
Makes 10 servings

1 c. chopped onion	1 c. cubed zucchini
2 T. olive oil	2 14.5 oz. cans tomatoes
1 c. diced carrot	3 c. water
1 c. minced celery	1 15 oz. can great northern beans, drained
1 t. oregano	¾ c. uncooked pasta
¼ t. pepper	¼ c. snipped fresh parsley
1 t. basil	

1. In a soup kettle, sauté onions in olive oil until they are soft, about 5 minutes.
2. Add carrot, celery, oregano, pepper, and basil. Cover and cook over low heat for 5 minutes.
3. Stir in zucchini, tomatoes, water, and beans. Cover and simmer gently for 30 minutes.
4. Heat soup to a boil.
5. Add pasta and boil until tender, about 10 minutes.
6. Stir in parsley and serve.

1. List five pieces of equipment you would need to prepare this recipe. <u>(List five:) dry measures, chef's knife, cutting board, measuring spoons, can opener, liquid measures, kitchen shears, soup kettle</u>

2. What do you need to do to the beans to get them ready to use? <u>Drain them.</u>

3. What do the abbreviations used with each of the following ingredients mean?

    A. onion <u>cup</u>   C. pepper <u>teaspoon</u>

    B. olive oil <u>tablespoon</u>   D. tomatoes <u>ounce</u>

4. Explain how the onions are to be cut. <u>into small pieces</u>

5. Explain how the carrots are to be cut. <u>into very small cubes of even size</u>

6. Explain how the celery is to be cut. <u>into very fine pieces</u>

7. Explain how the zucchini is to be cut. <u>into small squares of equal size</u>

8. Explain how the onions are to be cooked. <u>in a small amount of hot fat</u>

9. Explain the cooking term used in step 3. <u>to cook in liquid that is barely at the boiling point</u>

10. Explain the cooking term used in steps 4 and 5. <u>to cook in liquid at 212°F (100°C)</u>

11. If you figure that it would take 10 minutes to wash and cut all the vegetables, how much time would it take to prepare this recipe? <u>1 hour</u>

12. What is the yield of this recipe? <u>10 servings</u>

Food Preparation Crossword

Activity B

Chapter 12

Name _______________________

Date _______________________   Period _______________

Across

3. To cut into long, slender pieces.

6. To soak in a hot liquid.

9. To cook in the oven with dry heat.

10. To combine solid fat with flour using a pastry blender, two forks, or the fingers.

11. To soften solid fats, often by adding a second ingredient, such as sugar, and working with a wooden spoon or an electric mixer until the fat is creamy.

13. To cook in a small amount of hot fat.

14. To cut or break into thin pieces.

17. To cook food in a small amount of hot fat.

18. To combine two or more ingredients into one mass.

19. To heat sugar until a brown color and characteristic flavor develop.

20. To cook one food or several foods together in a seasoned liquid for a long period.

(Continued)

22. To remove a substance from the surface of a liquid.

23. To divide into parts with a sharp utensil.

25. To cut into very small cubes of even size.

27. To remove the seed(s) of a fruit or vegetable.

28. To cut food into thin, stick-sized strips.

32. To remove one part from another, as the yolk from the white of an egg.

33. To cut into small bits with kitchen shears.

37. To coat a food by sprinkling it with or dipping it in a dry ingredient such as flour or bread crumbs.

38. To shape by hand or by pouring into a form to achieve a desired structure.

39. To remove the center part of a fruit such as an apple or pineapple.

40. To leave an opening through which steam can escape in the covering of a food to be cooked in a microwave oven.

41. To put through a sieve to reduce to finer particles.

43. To make small, shallow cuts on the surface of a food.

44. To remove from a form.

46. To lift a food off the floor of a microwave oven to allow microwaves to penetrate the food from the bottom as well as from the top and sides.

Down

1. To make grooves or folds in dough.

2. To reduce a food into small bits by rubbing it on the sharp teeth of a utensil.

4. To quickly plunge blanched vegetables in cold water to stop the cooking process.

5. To return to a previous state by adding water.

6. To cook with vapor produced by a boiling liquid.

7. To put food through a fine sieve or a food mill to form a thick and smooth liquid.

8. To cut into four equal pieces.

10. To pulverize.

12. To soak meat in a solution containing an acid, such as vinegar or tomato juice, that helps tenderize the connective tissue.

15. To flatten dough to an even thickness with a rolling pin.

16. To prepare a food for cooking.

19. To mix or blend two or more ingredients.

21. To beat quickly and steadily by hand with a whisk or rotary beater.

24. To prepare fowl for cooking by binding the wings and legs.

25. To cause a solid food to turn into or become part of a liquid.

26. To work dough by pressing it with the heels of the hand, folding it, turning it, and repeating each motion until the dough is smooth and elastic.

29. To scatter drops of liquid or particles of powder over the surface of a food.

30. To cook on a rack or spit over hot coals or some other source of direct heat.

31. To rub fat on the surface of a cooking utensil or on a food itself.

34. To boil in liquid until partially cooked.

35. To mix ingredients together with a circular up and down motion using a spoon, whisk, or rotary or electric beater.

36. To remove bones from fowl or meat.

42. To incorporate a delicate mixture into a thicker, heavier mixture with a whisk or flexible spatula using a down, up, and over motion so the finished product remains light.

45. To place small pieces of butter or another food over the surface of a food.

Microwave Cooking

Activity C   **Name** _______________________________________

Chapter 12   **Date** _____________________________ **Period** _____________

Read the following scenarios about microwave cooking problems and answer the questions that follow in the space provided.

1. Carl put a frozen burrito in the microwave oven for three minutes. The burrito was steaming when Carl took it out of the oven, and he burned his tongue on the first bite. When Carl cut into the middle of the burrito, however, there were still ice crystals in the center. Why wasn't Carl's burrito hot all the way through?

   (Answers will vary.) ____

   ____

   How could Carl have helped the burrito heat more evenly? (Answers will vary.) __________

   ____

   ____

2. Jason's mother told him a medium-sized potato could be baked in the microwave oven in four minutes. When Jason cooked a potato for four minutes and then cut into it, it was raw in the center. What did Jason's mother forget to mention about microwaving potatoes that kept his from being fully cooked?

   (Answers will vary.) ____

   ____

   ____

3. Stephanie baked some brownies in the microwave oven in a square glass baking dish. When she cut the brownies, Stephanie discovered the ones in the middle of the pan were moist and chewy. However, the ones in the corners were hard and dry. What caused Stephanie's brownies to be hard in the corners?

   (Answers will vary.) ____

   ____

   How could she have prevented this from happening? (Answers will vary.) _____________

   ____

   ____

4. Manuel tightly covered a vegetable tray with plastic wrap before putting it in the microwave oven. Two minutes later, he looked through the window of the oven door. Manuel was surprised to see the wrap had formed a huge bubble over the tray. What caused the plastic wrap to form a bubble and how could this be prevented?

   (Answers will vary.) ____

   ____

   How should Manuel remove the wrap to avoid getting burned? (Answers will vary.) ______

   ____

   ____

      Copyright by Goodheart-Willcox Co., Inc.

Changing Recipe Yield

Activity D   **Name** ____

Chapter 12   **Date** _______________________________ **Period** _____________

In the spaces provided, write the yield and amounts of ingredients for a half recipe and a double recipe. Keep all measurements in the same units shown in the recipe. Then answer the questions that follow.

Half Recipe	**Turkey Joes**	**Double Recipe**
1. Serves 3 to 4	Serves 6 to 8	11. Serves 12 to 16
2. ¾ pound	1½ pounds ground turkey	12. 3 pounds
3. ¼ cup	½ cup chopped onion	13. 1 cup
4. ½ tablespoon	1 tablespoon flour	14. 2 tablespoons
5. 1 teaspoon	2 teaspoons brown sugar	15. 4 teaspoons
6. ½ teaspoon	1 teaspoon ground mustard	16. 2 teaspoons
7. ¾ teaspoon	1½ teaspoons chili powder	17. 3 teaspoons
8. ⅙ cup	⅓ cup water	18. ⅔ cup
9. 1 tablespoon	2 tablespoons cider vinegar	19. 4 tablespoons
10. ¾ cup	1½ cups chili sauce	20. 3 cups

21. How would you measure the amount of flour needed for half a recipe? 1½ teaspoons

22. How would you measure the amount of water needed for half a recipe? 2 tablespoons plus 2 teaspoons

23. Convert the amount of brown sugar needed for a double recipe into units that would require the least amount of measuring. 1 tablespoon plus 1 teaspoon

24. Convert the amount of chili powder needed for a double recipe into units that would require the least amount of measuring. 1 tablespoon

25. Convert the amount of vinegar needed for a double recipe into units that would require the least amount of measuring. ¼ cup

26. What is the metric equivalent of the amount of onion needed for half a recipe? 50 mL

27. What is the metric equivalent of the amount of mustard needed for half a recipe? 2 mL

28. What is the metric equivalent of the amount of vinegar needed for half a recipe? 15 mL

29. What is the metric equivalent of the amount of chili sauce needed for half a recipe? 175 mL

30. What is the metric equivalent of the amount of mustard needed for a single recipe? 5 mL

31. What is the metric equivalent of the amount of water needed for a single recipe? 75 mL

32. What is the metric equivalent of the amount of onion needed for a double recipe? 250 mL

33. What is the metric equivalent of the amount of water needed for a double recipe? 150 mL

34. What is the metric equivalent of the amount of vinegar needed for a double recipe? 50 mL

Making a Time-Work Schedule

Activity E   **Name** ____

Chapter 12   **Date** _________________________________ **Period** ______________

Plan a menu for a nutritious meal and make a time-work schedule for preparing it by following these steps:
1. List your menu items in the first column of the *Food Preparation Time Chart*.
2. Fill in your estimates for the time required for preparing, cooking, and serving each menu item.
3. Add the total time required to prepare each item.
4. In the last column of the chart, rank the menu items in order of the total time required to prepare them, with 1 requiring the most time.
5. Use the information in the *Food Preparation Time Chart* to complete the Time-Work Schedule. List the most important preparation tasks and specific times for completing them. Remember to allow your schedule to be flexible.

Food Preparation Time Chart

Menu Item	Preparation Time	Cooking Time	Serving Time	Total Time	Rank
(Chart answers will vary.)					
Table setting			10	10	

Time-Work Schedule

Time	Tasks

Create a Sandwich

Activity F   Name ____

Chapter 12   Date _______________________   Period __________

Circle a type of bread and one or more items from each of the other categories that follow to create a sandwich. Then name and describe your creation.

Breads	**Protein Fillings**	**Toppings**	**Spreads**
bagel	cheese	bacon bits	butter or margarine
French	chicken or turkey	green pepper	horseradish
Italian	ham	hot peppers	jelly
pita	hard-cooked egg	lettuce	ketchup
potato	luncheon meat	onion	mayonnaise
pumpernickel	peanut butter	pickles	mustard
raisin	roast beef	ripe olives	pickle relish
rye	tuna	shredded carrots	other______________
tortilla	other______________	spiced fruits	
whole wheat		tomatoes	
other______________		other______________	

What is the name of your sandwich creation? (Answers will vary.) _______________________

What made you choose the particular combination of ingredients you circled above? (Answers will vary.) __

____

Would you choose to serve this sandwich hot or cold? (Answers will vary.) ____________________

Answer the following questions about preparing sandwiches by circling *T* if the statement is true or *F* if the statement is false.

T (F)   1. Sandwich recipes tend to be complex.

(T) F   2. Sandwiches are popular for many events because they travel well, can be eaten without utensils, and are convenient to serve to groups.

T (F)   3. Sandwiches should be made on sandwich bread.

T (F)   4. Sandwich fillings are often dairy foods.

T (F)   5. Leaving sandwiches whole makes them easier to eat.

(T) F   6. Garnishes can improve the appearance and food value of sandwiches.

(T) F   7. Sandwiches should be kept refrigerated until serving time to prevent the growth of harmful bacteria.

(T) F   8. When packing sandwiches, chilled drinks can be used to keep perishable ingredients safe.

T (F)   9. Lettuce, tomato, and pickles should be put on sandwiches well before serving to allow flavors to blend.

T (F) 10. Hot sandwiches should be allowed to cool to room temperature before serving to prevent diners from burning their mouths on hot ingredients.

Snack and Beverage Survey

Activity G **Name** ___________________________________

Chapter 12 **Date** _____________________________ **Period** _____________

Survey five teens about their snack and beverage consumption habits. Record their answers in the table that follows the survey questions. Compile your results with those of your classmates. Write an article for your school paper reporting your findings. (Articles will vary.)

1. What is your gender?   A. male   B. female

2. When are you most likely to eat a snack?   A. midmorning   B. after school   C. at night

3. Which of the following would you be most likely to choose for a snack?   A. yogurt   B. chips
   C. cookies   D. cheese and crackers   E. fruit   F. carrot and celery sticks

4. Which factor is most important to you when choosing snack foods?   A. taste   B. nutrition
   C. convenience

5. Which of the following would you be most likely to choose for a cold drink?   A. milk   B. water
   C. regular carbonated beverage   D. diet beverage   E. fruit or vegetable juice   F. lemonade or fruit
   punch   G. smoothie or milk shake

6. Which type of coffee beverage would you be most likely to choose?   A. unflavored hot coffee
   B. flavored hot coffee   C. specialty hot coffee, such as cappuccino or latte   D. iced coffee drink
   E. I do not drink coffee.

7. Which type of tea do you prefer?   A. black   B. green   C. oolong   D. white   E. herbal   F. I do not
   drink tea.

8. Which type of coffee and/or tea do you prefer?   A. regular   B. decaffeinated

9. Why do you most often choose a snack or beverage?   A. to satisfy hunger or thirst   B. to socialize
   with friends   C. habit

10. How much money would you estimate spending each week on snacks and/or beverages?   A. under $5
    B. $5 to $10   C. $11 to $15   D. $16 to $20   E. over $20

Question	Teen #1	Teen #2	Teen #3	Teen #4	Teen #5
1	(Chart answers will vary.)				
2					
3					
4					
5					
6					
7					
8					
9					
10					

Grain Foods

Grains and Grain Products

Activity A Name _______________________________

Chapter 13 Date _____________________ Period ___________

1. Label and describe the three main parts of this kernel of grain.

A. <u>endosperm: contains most of the starch and protein of the kernel and holds the food supply the plant uses to grow</u>

B. <u>bran: the outer protective covering of the kernel, which is a good source of vitamins and fiber</u>

C. <u>germ: the reproductive part of the plant, rich in vitamins, minerals, protein, and fat</u>

Name the most important grains used for food in the United States by unscrambling the letters and writing the correct terms in the blanks.

2. H A T E W <u>W H E A T</u>

3. R O N C <u>C O R N</u>

4. L A E Y B R <u>B A R L E Y</u>

5. A T O S <u>O A T S</u>

6. I R E C <u>R I C E</u>

7. Y R E <u>R Y E</u>

Match the following descriptive phrases with the correct terms. Write your answer in the space provided to the left of the number.

<u>A</u> 8. A flour made from a blend of different varieties of wheat that is used for general cooking and baking.

<u>C</u> 9. A flour made from soft wheat that is used for cakes and other baked products with delicate textures.

<u>J</u> 10. A flour made from the entire wheat kernel that gives baked products a nutlike flavor and coarse texture.

<u>H</u> 11. Macaroni, noodles, and spaghetti.

<u>E</u> 12. Cereal products to which thiamin, niacin, riboflavin, folic acid, and iron have been added to replace nutrients lost due to processing.

<u>K</u> 13. The seed of a grass that grows in the marshes of Minnesota and Canada.

<u>G</u> 14. Corn minus the hull and germ.

<u>D</u> 15. The refined starch from the endosperm of corn.

<u>B</u> 16. Whole wheat that has been cooked, dried, partly debranned, and cracked.

<u>F</u> 17. A wheat product made by grinding and sifting wheat from which the bran and most of the germ has been removed.

A. all-purpose flour
B. bulgar wheat
C. cake flour
D. cornstarch
E. enriched
F. farina
G. hominy
H. pasta
I. pearl barley
J. whole wheat flour
K. wild rice

Breakfast Cereal Comparison

Activity B   **Name** ____

Chapter 13   **Date** _________________________ **Period** ____________

Record information from the Nutrition Facts panel of your choice of two ready-to-eat breakfast cereals in the spaces provided. Then answer the questions on the next page. (Chart answers will vary.)

Cereal A:	Cereal B:
Price:	Price:
Servings per container:	Servings per container:
Nutrition information per serving without milk	
Serving size:	Serving size:
Calories:	Calories:
Calories from fat:	Calories from fat:
Total fat:	Total fat:
Saturated fat:	Saturated fat:
Trans fat:	*Trans* fat:
Cholesterol:	Cholesterol:
Sodium:	Sodium:
Total carbohydrate:	Total carbohydrate:
Dietary fiber:	Dietary fiber:
Sugars:	Sugars:
Protein:	Protein:
Percent Daily Value	
Total fat:	Total fat:
Saturated fat:	Saturated fat:
Cholesterol:	Cholesterol:
Sodium:	Sodium:
Total carbohydrate:	Total carbohydrate:
Dietary fiber:	Dietary fiber:
Vitamin A:	Vitamin A:
Vitamin C:	Vitamin C:
Calcium:	Calcium:
Iron:	Iron:
Other nutrients:	Other nutrients:
List the first five ingredients shown on each label	

(Continued)

1. Which cereal is the most economical? (Answers will vary.)

2. Which cereal is lowest in fat? (Answers will vary.)

3. Which cereal is lowest in sodium? (Answers will vary.)

4. Which cereal is lowest in sugars? (Answers will vary.)

5. Which cereal is highest in fiber? (Answers will vary.)

6. Which cereal is highest in vitamins and minerals? (Answers will vary.)

7. Which cereal is the best source of whole grains? (Answers will vary.)

8. Which cereal would you rank as most nutritious overall? Explain your answer. (Answers will vary.)

9. Which cereal would you rather eat? Explain your answer. (Answers will vary.)

10. What size portion of this cereal do you typically eat? (Answers will vary.)

    How many ounce-equivalents from the grains group of MyPlate is this? (Answers will vary.)

11. How does this portion size affect your evaluation of nutrition label information? (Answers will vary.)

12. What type of milk do you pour on your cereal? (Answers will vary.)

13. How does the milk affect the nutritive value of the cereal? (Answers will vary.)

14. How much, if any, sugar do you add to your cereal before eating it? (Answers will vary.)

15. How does added sugar affect the nutritive value of the cereal? (Answers will vary.)

Cooking Starches and Cereals

Name ___________________________________

Date _______________________   Period _____________

Read the following statements about starch and cereal cookery. Circle *T* if the statement is true. Circle *F* if the statement is false.

T **(F)** 1. Starch is a simple carbohydrate stored in animals.

T **(F)** 2. Cornstarch- and tapioca-thickened mixtures are opaque.

T **(F)** 3. All starches behave the same way during cooking.

T **(F)** 4. Granular starch is soluble in both hot and cold water.

(T) F 5. Dry heat causes starch to lose some of its thickening power.

(T) F 6. When starch granules are combined with liquid and heated, they absorb the liquid and swell.

T **(F)** 7. To prevent overcooking, starch mixtures should be removed from the heat as soon as gelatinization occurs.

(T) F 8. Gentle stirring during cooking will help keep starch mixtures smooth.

(T) F 9. Coating starch granules with fat will prevent lumping.

(T) F 10. The relative low cost and high energy value of cereals make them an important part of the diet.

(T) F 11. Cooking improves the digestibility of cereal products.

(T) F 12. Whole grain cereals will cook more quickly if they are first soaked to soften the bran.

(T) F 13. Cooking cereals at temperatures that are too hot can cause lumping and scorching.

T **(F)** 14. Cereals that are finely granulated or precooked will cook slower than cracked or whole grain cereals.

(T) F 15. Properly cooked rice is tender and fluffy.

T **(F)** 16. White rice, brown rice, and instant rice all cook in about the same amount of time.

T **(F)** 17. Pasta should be added to cold water.

(T) F 18. As the starch granules swell, pasta doubles in size.

T **(F)** 19. Pasta products should be rinsed after draining.

(T) F 20. When cooked in a microwave oven, rice and cereal should be allowed to stand a few minutes before serving.

Vegetables

Selecting and Storing Vegetables

Activity A   **Name** _______________________________________

Chapter 14   **Date** _____________________________   **Period** _______________

The following statements about selecting and storing vegetables are false. Rewrite them to make them true. Write your responses in the space provided.

1. MyPlate suggests teens eat 1 to 2 cups per day from the vegetable group.______________________
   MyPlate suggests teens eat 2½ to 4 cups per day from the vegetable group.

2. Broccoli and carrots are in the "other vegetables" subgroup. Broccoli is in the dark green vegetables
   subgroup. Carrots are in the red and orange vegetables subgroup.

3. When selecting vegetables, select those that are very large.______________________________
   When selecting vegetables, select those that are medium in size.

4. Fresh vegetables retain their quality for a long while, so keep large quantities on hand.
   Fresh vegetables lose quality and nutrients through prolonged storage, so buy only what you will use
   within a short time.

5. Vegetables that are in season are usually high in quality and, therefore, high in price. _____________
   Vegetables that are in season are usually high in quality and low in price.

6. Potatoes and hard-rind squash should be stored in the crisper or in plastic bags or containers.
   Potatoes and hard-rind squash should be stored in a cool, dark, dry place.

7. To save money when buying canned vegetables, choose reduced-price, dented cans. _____________
   Choose cans that are free from dents, bulges, and leaks. Choose house brands to save money.

8. Canned vegetables retain the appearance and flavor of fresh vegetables better than frozen and
   dried vegetables.
   Frozen vegetables retain the appearance and flavor of fresh vegetables better than canned and
   dried vegetables.

9. To be sure vegetables are solidly frozen, choose packages with a heavy layer of ice on them.
   Choose packages that are clean and solidly frozen. A heavy layer of ice on the package may
   indicate the vegetables thawed and refroze.

10. The most commonly purchased dried vegetables are onions, mushrooms, and potatoes.___________
    The most commonly purchased dried vegetables are legumes—peas, beans, and lentils.

Cooking Vegetables by Class

Activity B   **Name** _______________________________________

Chapter 14   **Date** _____________________   **Period** ____________

In each of the following items, identify the pigment that gives vegetables the specified color. Describe the cooking method generally recommended for cooking vegetables of that color. Then give an example of a vegetable in that color category.

1. Green pigment: _chlorophyll_

   Cooking method: _Cook green vegetables in a small amount of water for a short time. Cook uncovered for the first few minutes, then cover._

   Example _(Answers will vary.)_

2. Orange pigment: _carotene_

   Cooking method: _Cook most orange vegetables in a small amount of water with the pan covered._

   Example _(Answers will vary.)_

3. White pigment: _flavones_

   Cooking method: _Avoid overcooking to prevent undesirable color changes._

   Example _(Answers will vary.)_

4. Red pigment: _anthocyanin_

   Cooking method: _Cook most red vegetables in a small amount of water, with the pan lid on, just until tender._

   Example _(Answers will vary.)_

Place each of the following vegetables in the appropriate flavor category in the chart below. Then describe the cooking method generally recommended for cooking vegetables in that category.

beets   corn   parsnips
broccoli   green beans   peas
Brussels sprouts   leeks   spinach
cabbage (green)   onions   yellow turnips

5. Mildly Flavored Vegetables	6. Strongly Flavored Vegetables	7. Very Strongly Flavored Vegetables
peas, green beans, spinach, corn, beets, parsnips	cabbage, broccoli, Brussels sprouts, yellow turnips	leeks, onions
Cooking method: Cook most mildly flavored vegetables in a small amount of water, with the pan covered, for a short time.	Cooking method: Cover strongly flavored vegetables with water. Cook them in an uncovered pan for a short time.	Cooking method: Cover very strongly flavored vegetables with water. Cook them in an uncovered pan for a longer time.

The Vegetable Cook

Name ____

Date _______________________________ Period _____________

Presume you are the vegetable cook in the kitchen of a large hotel restaurant. Use chapter information to answer the questions about the following situations, which you might encounter. Write your answers in the space provided.

1. The executive chef asks you to avoid preparing strong-flavored vegetables that might overwhelm the subtle flavors of her entrees.

   A. What vegetables should you avoid? ____

   cabbage, broccoli, Brussels sprouts, turnips, rutabagas, onions, leeks

   B. What vegetables might you prepare instead? _______________________________

   peas, green beans, spinach, corn, beets, parsnips

2. The executive chef has given you the responsibility of purchasing vegetables. The vegetable wholesaler offers you a discount on very small vegetables, very large vegetables, and very large quantities of vegetables. Explain your response to each of these discount offers.

   A. small vegetables ____

   I'm not interested in buying small vegetables because they can be immature and lack flavor.

   B. large vegetables ____

   I'm not interested in buying large vegetables because they can be overmature and tough.

   C. large quantities I buy only as many vegetables as I can use within a short time because

   vegetables lose quality quickly.

3. In the large hotel kitchen, refrigerated storage space is at a premium. However, there is some space in a cool, dry, unrefrigerated storage room you can use. Which of your vegetables can you store in the storage room?

   onions, potatoes, hard-rind squash, eggplant, rutabagas, sweet potatoes

4. An assistant is helping you prepare raw vegetables for salads and garnishes. He fills a large stainless steel sink with water and dumps in heads of broccoli and cauliflower to soak. Explain your response to your assistant's preparation technique.

   Wash vegetables under cool running water. Do not allow vegetables to soak because soaking can cause the loss of water-soluble nutrients.

5. During the lunchtime rush, waiters bring several orders of green beans back to the kitchen. The waiters tell you customers are complaining the vegetables are mushy and have a strange color.

   A. What has caused these unappealing characteristics? The green beans are overcooked.

   B. How can you avoid this problem when preparing green beans to accompany the dinner entrees?

   Cook green beans in a small amount of water. Use a short cooking time and keep the pan lid off for the first few minutes of cooking. Then cover the pan and cook the green beans just until they are crisp-tender.

6. The executive chef is planning a special German menu to celebrate Oktoberfest. She wants you to prepare red cabbage to serve with the sauerbraten. She warns she will not serve your cabbage if you let it turn purple.

    A. What would cause red cabbage to turn purple? _______________________________

    An alkali present in some water can cause the red pigment in cabbage to turn purple.

    B. How could you avoid an undesirable color change when preparing red cabbage?_____________

    Adding a small amount of an acid such as vinegar or lemon juice to the cooking water will
    neutralize the alkali and keep the cabbage red.

7. The banquet manager tells you she has scheduled a group luncheon next Friday. When picking the menu, the group's chairperson selected grilled steak accompanied by broiled tomatoes. How will you prepare the tomatoes?

    Cut the tomatoes in half and brush the cut surfaces with oil or melted fat. Then place the tomatoes
    under the broiling unit and broil until tender, watching carefully to avoid overcooking.

8. The executive chef wants to expand the variety of side dishes offered with dinner entrees. However, she does not want you to have to order a wider variety of vegetables from your wholesaler. Current side dishes include steamed broccoli, baked potatoes, and glazed carrots. Suggest a different way of serving each type of vegetable.

    A. broccoli __(Answers will vary.)__

    B. potatoes __(Answers will vary.)__

    C. carrots __(Answers will vary.)__

Fruits

Fruit Scramble

Activity A Name _______________________________________

Chapter 15 Date ___________________________ Period ____________

Unscramble the following letters to spell out the names of fruits. Write your answers in the space provided in the chart. Then check the appropriate column to identify the classification of each fruit.

Fruits	Berries	Drupes	Pomes	Citrus Fruits	Melons	Tropical Fruits
1. ganrose = oranges				✓		
2. palpes = apples			✓			
3. sanbaan = bananas						✓
4. neippalsep = pineapples						✓
5. aptocenaul = cantaloupe					✓	
6. rebrebslieu = blueberries	✓					
7. wabreriestrs = strawberries	✓					
8. pergaftuir = grapefruit				✓		
9. sperag = grapes	✓					
10. yapaap = papaya						✓
11. itwirfkui = kiwifruit						✓
12. shercrie = cherries		✓				
13. yhweeond = honeydew					✓	
14. sapre = pears			✓			
15. gantrinsee = tangerines				✓		
16. coptairs = apricots		✓				
17. slomen = lemons				✓		
18. tnelwamero = watermelon					✓	
19. muslp = plums		✓				
20. chepsea = peaches		✓				
21. gifs = figs						✓
22. dovcaao = avocado						✓
23. snirrrbeeca = cranberries	✓					
24. semli = limes				✓		
25. acaabs = casaba					✓	

Mixed Fruit

Activity B   **Name** _______________________________________

Chapter 15   **Date** _______________________   **Period** ____________

Describe quality factors you should seek when selecting each of the following fruits in its specified form. Explain how to properly store each type of fruit. Then describe how to prepare the fruit for its specified use. If no use is specified, indicate how you would choose to serve the fruit and describe the preparation technique.

1. Fruit: frozen strawberries

   Use: (Answers will vary.)

   Selection: Packages should be clean, undamaged, and frozen solid.

   Storage: Store in the coldest part of the freezer. Store thawed, unused berries in a tightly covered container in the refrigerator.

   Preparation: (Answers will vary.)

2. Fruit: fresh bananas

   Use: fresh fruit salad

   Selection: Can be purchased when underripe (green). Avoid bruised or damaged fruit.

   Storage: Ripen at room temperature. Refrigerate ripened fruit.

   Preparation: Dip cut bananas in lemon, orange, grapefruit, or pineapple juice to prevent enzymatic browning and make them look more appealing.

3. Fruit: canned peaches

   Use: (Answers will vary.)

   Selection: Cans should be free from dents, bulges, and leaks.

   Storage: Store cans in a cool, dry place. Cover and refrigerate fruit after opening.

   Preparation: (Answers will vary.)

4. Fruit: raisins

   Use: cooked raisin sauce

   Selection: Fruit should be soft and pliable.

   Storage: Store unopened package in a cool, dark, dry place. After opening, store in tightly covered container.

   Preparation: Soak in hot water for about an hour before cooking to soften and rehydrate.

Dairy Products

Dairy Identification

Activity A   Name ____

Chapter 16   Date _______________________   Period ____________

Match the following descriptions with the dairy products they describe. Place the correct letters in the corresponding blanks to the left of each number.

___T___ 1. Fluid milk that must contain at least 3.25 percent milk fat and 8.25 percent milk solids.

___E___ 2. Fluid milk that has nearly all of the fat removed.

___F___ 3. Milk with added flavoring.

___I___ 4. Milk that has been treated with lactase to break down milk sugar.

___P___ 5. A nondairy product that is an alternative to fluid milk for lactose-intolerant people.

___H___ 6. The type of cream that has the most fat.

___L___ 7. A type of cream that will hold air when whipped but has less fat than heavy whipping cream.

___G___ 8. A product made from half milk and half cream.

___U___ 9. A cultured dairy product that may contain added nonfat milk solids and flavorings or fruits.

___B___ 10. A cultured dairy product used for cooking and baking as well as drinking.

___O___ 11. A cultured dairy product made from light cream.

___C___ 12. Sterilized, homogenized whole, reduced fat, or fat-free milk that has had some of the water removed.

___Q___ 13. Whole or fat-free milk with some of the water removed and a sweetener added.

___N___ 14. A product made by removing most of the water and fat from whole milk.

___J___ 15. A product that must show at least a 50 percent reduction in fat over regular ice cream.

___D___ 16. A frozen dairy dessert that must contain less than 0.5 grams of fat per serving.

___K___ 17. A product made from churned pasteurized cream, which is often preferred for use at the table and in cooking.

___R___ 18. A product made from churned pasteurized cream, which is often preferred for baking.

___S___ 19. A nondairy product that gets the body and appearance of whipped cream from substances such as soy protein, emulsifiers, and vegetable fats and gums.

___M___ 20. A nondairy product often used in place of butter.

A. coffee whitener
B. cultured buttermilk
C. evaporated milk
D. fat-free frozen yogurt
E. fat-free milk
F. flavored milk
G. half-and-half
H. heavy whipping cream
I. lactose-reduced milk
J. light ice cream
K. lightly salted butter
L. light whipping cream
M. margarine
N. nonfat dry milk
O. regular sour cream
P. soy milk
Q. sweetened condensed milk
R. unsalted butter
S. whipped topping
T. whole milk
U. yogurt

Buying and Storing Dairy Products

Activity B **Name** _______________________________

Chapter 16 **Date** _____________________ **Period** ____________

Underline the dairy products and foods containing dairy products in the menus that follow. Write a shopping list of all the dairy products you would need to buy to prepare these menus. Then plan a snack for each day using some of the leftover dairy products and answer the question at the bottom of the page.

	Day 1	Day 2
Breakfast	Scrambled Eggs Sausage Links Whole Wheat Toast Grapefruit Half Milk Coffee	Bagel Cream Cheese Orange Juice Chocolate Milk
Lunch	Grilled American Cheese Sandwiches Cream of Tomato Soup Tossed Salad Baked Apple Lemonade	Ham and Swiss Sandwiches Fruit Salad/Yogurt Dressing Sugar Cookies Cola
Dinner	Roast Beef Mashed Potatoes Broccoli Cheddar Cheese Sauce Cloverleaf Rolls Pumpkin Pie/Whipped Cream Milk	Broiled Fish Rice Pilaf Sauteed Asparagus Peach Half/Cottage Cheese Butter Pecan Ice Cream Iced Tea
Snack	(Answers will vary.) _______________ _______________ _______________	_______________ _______________ _______________ _______________

Shopping List

milk

American cheese

Cheddar cheese

whipping cream

cream cheese

chocolate milk

Swiss cheese

yogurt

cottage cheese

butter pecan ice cream

(Students may justify underlining additional menu items in which dairy products might be used.)

What are three tips for storing dairy products to help maintain their flavors and nutrients?

(Answers will vary.)

____

____

____

____

Cheese Tasting

<table>
<tr><td>Activity C</td><td>Name _______________________________________</td></tr>
<tr><td>Chapter 16</td><td>Date ___________________________ Period ____________</td></tr>
</table>

Sample a variety of cheeses. In the table that follows, list the kinds of cheese you sampled and describe their appearances, textures, and flavors. Then complete the items at the bottom of the page.

Variety of Cheese	Appearance	Texture	Flavor
Ripened cheese:	(Table answers will vary.)		
Ripened cheese:			
Ripened cheese:			
Unripened cheese:			
Unripened cheese:			
Process cheese:			
Imitation cheese:			

1. Describe how you would serve one of the above cheeses as an appetizer or snack. ______________
   (Answers will vary.)

2. Describe how you would serve one of the above cheeses in a sandwich. (Answers will vary.)
   ____

3. Describe how you would use one of the above cheeses in cooking. (Answers will vary.)
   ____

4. Describe how you would serve one of the above cheeses as part of a dessert. (Answers will vary.)
   ____

5. What is the best way to store cheese? Cover or tightly wrap and refrigerate it.
   ____

6. Besides maintaining wholesomeness, what are the benefits of storing cheese properly? __________
   Proper storage prevents cheese from becoming dry and prevents the spread of odors and flavors.

Cooking with Milk

Activity D   Name ____

Chapter 16   Date ____________________________   Period _____________

Undesirable reactions that can occur when cooking with milk are given below. Identify each problem by reading the clues. Then describe a method that could be used to prevent the undesirable reaction.

Problem 1. <u>curdling</u> Clumps have formed in a scalloped potato and ham casserole.	This problem can be prevented by <u>using low temperatures and fresh milk</u> ___________________________________ ___________________________________
Problem 2. <u>scum formation</u> A solid layer has formed on the surface of hot chocolate.	This problem can be prevented by <u>stirring the milk during heating, covering the</u> <u>pan, or beating the milk with a whisk or rotary</u> <u>beater to form a foam layer</u>
Problem 3. <u>scorching</u> Milk heated in a pan has a brown color and a coating has formed on the bottom of the pan.	This problem can be prevented by <u>using low heat or by heating the milk in the top</u> <u>of a double boiler</u> ___________________________________

The steps for preparing a white sauce using a slurry and a roux are listed in two groups below. Read the steps in each group. Reorganize them in the correct order by placing the letters of the corresponding steps in the blanks. When completed, the letters will spell out the name of a white sauce recipe variation.

1. ____C____   M __5__ Cook the slurry for one minute longer until the sauce is smooth and thickened.

2. ____R____   C __1__ Combine fat-free milk, flour, and seasonings in a blender container or small, covered jar.

3. ____E____   E __3__ Cook the slurry in a heavy saucepan over medium heat.

4. ____A____   R __2__ Blend or shake until thoroughly mixed.

5. ____M____   A __4__ Stir gently until the mixture reaches a boil.

6. ____S____   U __8__ Stir milk into the roux.

7. ____O____   O __7__ Stir in flour and seasonings to form a paste.

8. ____U____   P __9__ Stir constantly while cooking the mixture over medium heat until it thickens into a smooth sauce.

9. ____P____   S __6__ Melt the fat over low heat.

10. List three uses of white sauce in cooking.

   A. <u>(List three:) a base for other sauces, cream soups, creamed vegetables and meats, soufflés,</u>

   B. <u>croquettes</u> ____

   C. ____

The Dairy Barn

Activity E　　　　Name ____

Chapter 16　　　　Date __________________________　　Period ____________

Presume you are the cook at a small family-owned restaurant called *The Dairy Barn*. This quaint country restaurant features dairy products from local farms in nearly all its dishes. Use chapter information to describe how you would handle each of the following situations involving preparing foods with dairy ingredients.

1. One of your most popular desserts is cheesecake made with cream cheese and sour cream. What ingredient substitutions can you make in your recipe to prepare a low-fat version of this dessert?

   Use reduced-fat cream cheese in place of regular cream cheese and plain, nonfat yogurt in place of sour cream.

2. The owner's son, Josh, often helps you in the kitchen when he's not busy with farm chores. Josh is a good worker but does not have a lot of cooking experience. This morning, you asked Josh to heat a pan of milk to make hot chocolate for the breakfast crowd. When you returned to check on Josh about 15 minutes later, you found him staring at a large puddle of milk covering the cooktop around the pan.

   A. What probably caused Josh's problem? *Scum formation on the surface of the milk probably caused pressure to build up until the milk boiled over.*

   B. What do you need to tell Josh to do to prevent this problem in the future? *Use low heat and stir milk during heating, cover the pan, or beat the milk with a whisk or rotary beater to form a foam layer.*

3. Josh needs to start over with the hot chocolate. He fills a bowl with milk and puts it in the microwave oven to heat while he cleans the mess on the cooktop. He's just about to press the button for high power when you stop him. What advice do you need to give Josh about microwaving milk?

   Use lower settings when microwaving milk to prevent curdling. Fill the bowl no more than two-thirds full to prevent boiling over.

4. After the breakfast rush, you begin working on some preparations for lunch. One task on your list is to whip some cream to serve on the desserts. You spend 20 minutes trying to whip the cream without success. Then you realize that what you thought was light whipping cream is actually labeled *light cream*.

   A. Why were you having trouble whipping this product? *Cream must contain at least 25 percent milk fat to whip successfully.*

   B. Josh watches as you start your task over, this time using the right type of cream. He wants to know why you are using a mixing bowl and beaters that you have just taken from the walk-in refrigerator. What do you tell him?

   For best results when whipping cream, thoroughly chill the bowl, beaters, and cream.

5. One of The Dairy Barn's most popular entrees is roast beef with mashed potatoes and creamy brown gravy. You prepared the roast beef earlier. Now, while you get started on the mashed potatoes, you ask Josh to work on the brown gravy. You showed him how to make a basic white sauce last week. What additional instructions do you need to give him about how to make gravy?

   Juice from meat or poultry are used in place of some or all of the milk in white sauce to give gravy flavor.

(Continued)

　　　　

6. Cream soups always go over well with your lunch patrons. You prepared enough cream of mushroom soup yesterday to serve again today.

    A. What will you need to remember when reheating it? ___________________________________

    Use low heat when reheating cream soup to prevent scorching.

    B. In addition to the cream of mushroom, you are preparing corn chowder for today's menu. You've cooked the potatoes, onions, and corn in chicken stock until tender. What do you need to remember now as you add the milk?

    Add the milk slowly and stir gently until blended. Heat at a low temperature to prevent curdling.

7. One of the desserts on today's lunch menu is chocolate pudding.

    A. What do you have to remember when stirring eggs into the pudding?

    Add a small amount of the hot pudding to the beaten eggs and then add the diluted egg mixture
    to the rest of the hot pudding.

    B. How can you prevent a skin from forming on the surface of the pudding as it cools?

    Place a piece of waxed paper on the surface of the warm pudding.

8. Although The Dairy Barn has a number of tasty desserts on the menu, the best seller is definitely the homemade ice cream. Unfortunately, the motor burned out on your ice cream freezer and you won't be able to get a replacement for a few days. In the meantime, you will have to make the ice cream using your walk-in freezer.

    A. Why are you concerned that making the ice cream this way might cause it to taste grainy?

    In the walk-in freezer, the ice cream will not be stirred continuously, so larger ice crystals can
    form. Frozen desserts that have large ice crystals taste grainy.

    B. What can you do to help give your ice cream the creamy taste your customers have grown to love?

    Add cooked beaten egg whites, whipped cream, whipped evaporated milk, or whipped gelatin to
    the recipe to inhibit the formation of ice crystals.

9. You originally offered macaroni and cheese on the kids' menu. However, adults liked it so much that you soon added it to the regular menu, too.

    A. How do you prepare the cheese to help it blend quickly into the creamy cheese sauce?

    Grating or shredding the cheese will help it blend more quickly than leaving it in large
    chunks.

    B. Why did you decide to use process cheese in this recipe instead of natural cheese?

    Process cheese blends more easily than natural cheese because of the emulsifiers it contains.

10. Your special blend of seasonings and sharp Cheddar produced at a local farm are the reason your cheese toast appetizers appear on nearly every dinner order. How do you need to melt the cheese under the broiler?

    Place the appetizers four or five inches from the heat, watch them carefully, and remove them
    when the cheese has melted.

Eggs

Selecting and Storing Eggs

Activity A **Name** ______________________________________

Chapter 17 **Date** _____________________ **Period** ____________

Complete the following items related to the selection and storage of eggs. Write your responses in the space provided.

Fill-in-the-Blanks: Complete the following statements by filling in the blanks.

1. Eggs are one of the best food sources of ______complete protein______.

2. Because egg yolks are high in ______cholesterol______, many health experts recommend using egg yolks and whole eggs in moderation.

3. Eggs are graded for quality by a system called ______candling______.

4. The grades of eggs available in most supermarkets are U.S. Grade ______AA and A______.

5. Most recipes are formulated to use ______large______ size eggs.

Identification:

6. From the list below, check the four quality factors that describe Grade AA and Grade A eggs.

__✓__ A. clean, unbroken shells ______ E. thin egg whites

__✓__ B. firm yolks ______ F. large size

______ C. large air cells __✓__ G. small air cells

______ D. unbroken shells that may be slightly stained __✓__ H. thick, clear egg whites

Short Answer: Answer the following questions to show your understanding.

7. What two factors affect variation in egg prices? grade and egg size

8. What size eggs do most shoppers buy? large

9. How many eggs would it take to equal a three-ounce portion of lean, cooked meat? three

10. Why are Grade B eggs rarely seen in food stores? because they are usually used in other food products

11. How are egg sizes determined? Eggs are sized on the basis of an average weight per dozen.

12. Why is it important to avoid buying cracked eggs? Cracked eggs can contain harmful bacteria, which can cause foodborne illness.

13. How should eggs be stored in the refrigerator? Eggs should be stored in their original carton, large end up.

14. How long can eggs be safely stored in a refrigerator? three to five weeks

15. How should leftover egg yolks and egg whites be stored?

    Yolks: Cover yolks with cold water and refrigerate in a tightly covered container.

    Whites: Refrigerate whites in a tightly covered container.

Functions of Eggs

Name _______________________________

Date _______________________________   Period _______________

The main functions performed by eggs in recipes are listed in the following chart. Describe these functions and give an example of a food product in which each function is performed. Write your responses in the space provided.

Function	Description	Food product
Nutrient additive	Eggs contribute important nutrients to food products.	(Food products are student response.)
Flavoring additive	Eggs affect the tastes of food products.	
Coloring agent	Eggs give an appealing color to some food products.	
Structure agent	Coagulated egg proteins create a framework around air cells in baked goods.	
Thickener	Heat causes egg proteins to coagulate, which adds thickness to foods containing eggs.	
Binding agent	Eggs hold together ingredients in foods.	
Interfering agent	Eggs interfere with the formation of large ice crystals, which would ruin the texture of frozen desserts.	
Foam	Air cells formed when air is beaten into egg whites and add air to foods.	
Emulsifier	Egg yolk keeps oil droplets suspended in a water-based liquid so the two liquids will not separate.	

Egg Dishes

Name ____

Date _________________________________ **Period** ______________

Place the specified letter in the blank to the left of each number to indicate whether each of the following statements is *true* or *false*. When completed, the letters will spell out a term related to the chapter.

E (true) _______ 1. Temperature, time, and the addition of other ingredients affect egg coagulation. (E = true; M = false)

M (false) _______ 2. High temperatures are recommended for egg cookery. (G = true; M = false)

U (true) _______ 3. When frying an egg, covering the skillet will cause the upper surface of the egg to cook. (U = true; O = false)

L (false) _______ 4. Scrambled eggs should be stirred constantly during cooking. (G = true; L = false)

S (true) _______ 5. When poaching eggs, a small amount of vinegar added to the cooking water will keep the egg whites from spreading. (S = true; C = false)

I (true) _______ 6. When baking eggs, individual baking dishes should be placed in a shallow casserole filled with 1 inch of warm water. (I = true; O = false)

F (false) _______ 7. Soft-cooked eggs are boiled in water for one to two minutes. (K = true; F = false)

Y (false) _______ 8. A greenish-colored ring around the yolk of a hard-cooked egg is toxic and should not be eaten. (E = true; Y = false)

I (false) _______ 9. Egg substitutes are made largely from soy protein. (R = true; I = false)

N (true) _______ 10. When making a puffy omelet, the egg yolks and egg whites are beaten separately and then folded together. (N = true; Y = false)

G (false) _______ 11. Soufflés should be allowed to stand 10 to 15 minutes after being removed from the oven. (M = true; G = false)

A (false) _______ 12. Beading is the leakage of liquid from a gel that sometimes occurs between a meringue and a pie filling. (E = true; A = false)

G (false) _______ 13. Hard meringues contain a lower proportion of sugar than soft meringues. (T = true; G = false)

E (true) _______ 14. Soft custards are stirred more than baked custards. (E = true; H = false)

N (false) _______ 15. The use of low heat can cause soft custard to curdle. (O = true; N = false)

T (true) _______ 16. A baked custard is done if the tip of a knife inserted into the center comes out clean. (T = true; D = false)

Term spelled out: ___(Correct answer spells *emulsifying agent*.)___________________

Scrambled Eggs

Name ___________________________________

Date _______________________ Period ____________

Unscramble the words below. Then write the letters of the correct words in the blanks to complete the following statements about eggs.

A. ACNPHIGO   P O A C H I N G

B. GFLINOD   F O L D I N G

C. OESLUFF   S O U F F L É

D. IWEPEGN   W E E P I N G

E. CTASUDR   C U S T A R D

F. GTINFIEERRN NEATG   I N T E R F E R I N G   A G E N T

G. AIEGBND   B E A D I N G

H. NOIELSMU   E M U L S I O N

I. SSEENSRIY   S Y N E R E S I S

J. IEMRTENPG   T E M P E R I N G

K. SREIRHD   S H I R R E D

L. NRIUMEGE   M E R I N G U E

M. LEEOTM   O M E L E T

N. GUUCLOMA   C O A G U L U M

O. FITSF AEKP   S T I F F   P E A K

1. Warming eggs to keep them from forming lumps when adding them to a hot mixture is called __J__.

2. Eggs act as an __F__ in some frozen desserts by inhibiting the formation of large ice crystals.

3. When egg whites are beaten to the __O__ stage, the peaks stand up straight.

4. The blending process used to avoid a loss of air when combining egg white foams with other ingredients is known as __B__.

5. Eggs are used to form a permanent __H__ in mayonnaise.

6. When heat is applied to eggs, they form soft protein clumps, which are called __N__.

7. __A__ is done by slipping an egg into a saucepan filled with 2 to 3 inches of simmering liquid.

8. Baked eggs are also called __K__ eggs.

9. A puffy __M__ is baked in a preheated oven.

10. A __C__ is a light, airy egg dish that can be served as a dessert or a main dish, depending on the added ingredients.

11. A hard __L__ may be used as a dessert base.

12. The layer of moisture that sometimes forms between a meringue and a pie filling is known as __D__.

13. Golden droplets that appear on the surface of a meringue are known as __G__.

14. A mixture of milk, eggs, sugar, and a flavoring that is cooked until thickened is a __E__.

15. Custards are baked in a pan of warm water to help prevent __I__.

Meat

The Meat Case

Activity A   Name ____

Chapter 18   Date ____________________   Period ____________

Use the following clues to help you identify items you might see in a supermarket meat case. Write your answers in the blanks to the left of each number.

______*meat*______ 1. The edible portions of mammals are called ______.

______*variety meats*______ 2. The edible parts of an animal other than the muscles are called ______.

______*proteins*______ 3. All meat and meat products provide ______, which are needed to build and repair tissue.

______*fat*______ 4. Ground meats are generally higher in ______ than all other cuts.

______*beef*______ 5. Meat that comes from mature cattle is called ______.

______*wholesale cuts*______ 6. Animal carcasses are divided into smaller pieces called ______ for easier handling by meat cutters.

______*retail cuts*______ 7. At the grocery store, meat cutters divide meats into smaller pieces called ______.

______*hamburger*______ 8. A ground beef product that can have extra fat added to it during grinding is called ______.

______*veal*______ 9. Meat that comes from young calves is called ______.

______*pork*______ 10. The meat of swine is called ______.

______*ham*______ 11. Cured, smoked meat from a pork leg is sold as ______.

______*bacon*______ 12. Smoked pork belly meat is known as ______.

______*lamb*______ 13. The meat of sheep less than one year old is sold as ______.

______*mutton*______ 14. The meat from sheep over two years of age is called ______.

______*inspection*______ 15. A round, purple ______ stamp assures buyers of wholesale cuts that meat is wholesome.

______*graded*______ 16. Animal carcasses may be voluntarily ______ for quality.

______*USDA*______ 17. The voluntary meat grading program is overseen by the ______.

______*marbling*______ 18. Flecks of fat throughout the lean muscles of meat are known as ______.

______*Choice and Select*______ 19. The most common grades of beef sold in retail stores are ______.

______*Prime*______ 20. Fine restaurant menus often offer the highest beef grade, which is ______.

Tough or Tender?

Activity B **Name** ______________________________

Chapter 18 **Date** ___________________ **Period** ___________

Use Figure 18-2 on page 335 in the text to help you complete the following table. Identify the location in the animal of each beef wholesale cut. Indicate whether cuts from this part of the animal are generally *tender* or *less tender*. List whether dry-heat or moist-heat cooking methods are generally recommended. In the last column, list two examples of retail cuts that come from this part of the animal. Then answer the questions at the bottom of the page. (Examples of retail cuts will vary. See Figure 18-2 on page 335 of the text.)

Wholesale Cut	A. Location in Animal	B. Tenderness	C. Cooking Method	D. Retail Cuts
1. Chuck	shoulder areas	less tender	moist heat	
2. Rib	back	tender	dry heat	
3. Loin	back	tender	dry heat	
4. Sirloin	hip	tender	dry heat	
5. Round	leg	less tender	moist heat	
6. Shank and brisket	arm and breast	less tender	moist heat	
7. Plate and flank	breast and side	less tender	moist heat	

8. What are the dry-heat cooking methods? roasting, broiling, grilling, panbroiling, frying

9. What are the moist-heat cooking methods? braising, cooking in liquid

10. How can less tender cuts be successfully cooked with a dry-heat method? Dry-heat methods can be successfully used with less tender cuts that have been mechanically or chemically tenderized.

Buying and Storing Meat

Activity C   Name ______________________________

Chapter 18   Date ___________________   Period ___________

In the space provided, complete the following exercises about buying and storing meat.

Reading a Meat Label

Use the meat label to answer questions about the piece of meat on which the label would appear.

1. What is the wholesale cut from which this piece of meat comes? _round_

2. What is the name of the retail cut of this piece of meat? _boneless top roast_

3. How much does this piece of meat weigh? _3.18 pounds_

4. What is the unit price of this meat? _$5.99 per pound_

5. How much would you have to pay for this piece of meat? _$19.05_

MEAT DEPARTMENT		
WEIGHT Lb. Net 3.18	PAY $19.05	PRICE Per Lb. 5.99
BEEF ROUND BONELESS TOP ROAST		

Deciding How Much to Buy

Use text information about the number of servings per pound provided by meat cuts with various bone content to answer the questions below.

6. How many servings would you get from a boneless ham weighing 4.6 pounds? _14 to 18 servings_

7. How many pounds of spare ribs would you need to buy for a picnic at which you expect 12 people? _6 to 9 pounds_

8. How much roast beef would you need to buy to serve six people for dinner and have enough leftovers to make four sandwiches for lunch the next day? _3 to 5 pounds_

9. How many patties should you be able to get from a package of ground chuck weighing 1.8 pounds? _5 to 7 patties_

10. Will you get more servings from 2.5 pounds of bone-in pork chops or 1.9 pounds of boneless chops? Explain your answer. _Boneless chops offer more servings per pound due to less waste._

Figuring Cost per Serving

Use text information about the number of servings per pound provided by various meat cuts to calculate the cost per serving in each of the following problems.

11. Baby back ribs are on sale for $3.99 a pound. _$2.00 to $2.99 per serving_

12. Boneless chuck roast for $4.99 a pound. _$1.25 to $1.66 per serving_

13. Lamb loin chops for $12.99 a pound. _$4.33 to $6.50 per serving_

14. Strip steak for $11.99 a pound. _$4.00 to $6.00 per serving_

15. Which is the better buy—8-bone pork roast for $4.99 a pound or boneless center loin pork roast for $5.49 a pound? Explain your answer. _Boneless roast yields more servings per pound for lower cost per serving._

Storing Meat

Answer the following questions about storing meat.

16. How should canned ham be stored? _Refrigerate it until ready to use unless the label says otherwise._

17. In what part of the refrigerator should meat be stored? _in coldest part of the refrigerator_

18. How should prepackaged meat be wrapped for refrigerator storage? _in its original wrapper_

19. How should meats be wrapped for extended freezer storage? _Rewrap it in moistureproof and vaporproof paper._

20. At what temperature should the refrigerator and freezer be set? _refrigerator 40°F or less/freezer 0°_

Cooking Meats

Name _______________________________

Date _____________________________   Period ____________

Match each of the following statements with the meat cooking method it describes by placing the correct letter in the space provided to the left of each number. Then answer the questions that follow.

____H____ 1. Place meat with the fat side up on a rack in a large, shallow pan. Meat is cooked, uncovered, in a slow oven until it reaches the desired degree of doneness.

____B____ 2. Meat is cooked, one side at a time, under a direct heat source.

____E____ 3. Remove heat source under the center of the cooking surface, where meat is placed. Cover to surround meat with heat and cook without turning until meat is done.

____G____ 4. Meat is cooked, uncovered, in a heavy skillet or griddle without using fat.

____D____ 5. Meat is cooked in a small amount of fat or in deep fat.

____A____ 6. Meat is browned slowly, and then it is cooked in a small amount of liquid over low heat.

____C____ 7. Meat is covered with water or stock. The kettle is covered, and the meat is allowed to simmer until it is tender.

A. braising
B. broiling
C. cooking in liquid
D. frying
E. grilling
F. microwaving
G. panbroiling
H. roasting

8. What are the recommended time frames during which refrigerated meats should be cooked or frozen?
1 to 2 days for ground meats, 3 to 4 days for nonground products, 3 days for leftovers

9. What are the food safety guidelines regarding marinade used for raw meat? _______________
Discard it or boil it for 1 minute before using it on cooked meat.

10. What are the safe internal temperatures for cooked meats? _______________
ground meats—160°F (70°C); beef and pork cuts—145°F (65°C)

11. How does a meat thermometer need to be handled after use?_______________
Wash the probe of a meat thermometer in hot, soapy water after each use.

12. Why should meats be covered when they are cooked in a microwave oven? _______________
Cover meats to keep them moist and tender and shorten the cooking time even further.

13. How can the appearance of meats cooked in a microwave oven be made more appealing?
A sauce or topping can be used to hide the lack of browning on meats cooked in a microwave oven.

14. What types of variety meats may be cooked by dry heat? _______________
brains, sweetbreads, and the liver and kidneys of young calves

15. Why is it recommended that meat not be thawed on the kitchen counter?_______________
Harmful microorganisms can grow that can result in foodborne illness.

16. When broiling, why place frozen meats farther away from the heat source than thawed meats?
This will prevent the outside from overcooking before the inside is cooked.

Poultry

Poultry Pointers

Activity A	**Name** _______________________________
Chapter 19	**Date** _________________ **Period** _________

Fill in the puzzle with words needed to complete the tips on poultry selection and storage given below.

```
                1. P  O U L T R Y
             2. G O   O  S E
        3. O U N C E - E Q  U  I V A L E N T S
             4. S E         L  F - B A S T I N G
             5. F A         T
             6. F           R  O Z E N
        7. Q U A L I T      Y

             8.  I N S  P  E C T E D
             9.  Y    O  U N G
            10.  L    I  G H T
            11. W I   N  G S
            12. M E A  T  Y
        13. F R E E Z  E  R  B U R N
        14. B A C T E  R  I A
            15. M O I  S  T U R E P R O O F
```

1. Any domesticated bird can be described as ______.

2. The types of poultry most commonly eaten in the United States are chicken, turkey, ______, and duck protein foods.

3. A small chicken breast half counts as 3 ______ from the protein foods group of MyPlate.

4. Poultry labeled as ______ is prepared with a solution that contains added sodium.

5. Turkey and chicken are lower in calories and total and saturated ______ than many cuts of red meat.

6. Poultry can be purchased fresh, ______, and in processed poultry products.

7. Poultry can be voluntarily graded for ______.

8. All poultry that is processed and sold as canned poultry is ______ for wholesomeness before canning.

9. Most fresh and frozen poultry is marketed ______, so the meat is tender and suitable for all cooking methods.

10. Breast meat is ______ and mildly flavored compared with dark meat.

11. Breasts, legs, and thighs are meatier than ______ and backs.

12. When buying poultry, choose birds with ______ breasts and legs, well-distributed fat, and blemish-free skin.

13. When buying frozen poultry beware of dirty and torn wrappers and pale, dry, frosty areas, which indicate ______. (two words)

14. Proper storage of poultry is important to inhibit the growth of salmonellae, an illness-causing ______.

15. For freezer storage, rewrap poultry in ______ and vaporproof wrapping and use within six to eight months.

Selecting and Storing Poultry

Name _______________________________

Date _______________________   Period ____________

Write the letter of the answer that *best* completes each statement in the space provided to the left of each number.

B 1. Dark meat is slightly ______ in fat than light meat.
    A. lower
    B. higher

B 2. A lot of the fat in poultry is located ______.
    A. throughout the muscle
    B. just under the skin

A 3. All poultry sold in interstate commerce must be federally ______ for wholesomeness.
    A. inspected
    B. graded

B 4. Dark meat has a ______ flavor than light meat.
    A. milder
    B. stronger

A 5. Chicken breasts, legs, and thighs are ______ than wings and backs.
    A. meatier
    B. less meaty

A 6. Poultry contains ______ bone in proportion to muscle than does red meat.
    A. more
    B. less

A 7. You need to allow about ______ of meat per serving when buying chicken.
    A. ½ pound
    B. ¾ pound

B 8. Ducks and geese have ______ meat.
    A. both light and dark
    B. all dark

A 9. Ducks and geese have ______ fat than chickens or turkeys.
    A. more
    B. less

A 10. Canned poultry items are generally ______ expensive than fresh-chilled or frozen poultry.
    A. more
    B. less

A 11. Poultry parts are ______ perishable than whole birds.
    A. more
    B. less

A 12. Wrap and store giblets ______ the rest of the bird.
    A. separately from
    B. with

A 13. Poultry can be stored in the freezer for ______.
    A. six to eight months
    B. up to one year

B 14. Frozen poultry that has thawed ______ be refrozen.
    A. can
    B. should not

Cooking Poultry

Activity C   **Name** _______________________________________

Chapter 19   **Date** _____________________ **Period** ___________

Answer the following questions about cooking poultry. Write your answers in the space provided.

1. What are the principles for cooking poultry and what happens when they are not followed?
   Poultry should be cooked at low temperatures using careful timing. Poultry that is cooked at too high a temperature or cooked too long is tough, dry, and flavorless.

2. How can you test poultry for doneness?
   A meat thermometer is the only accurate way to test poultry for doneness. Insert the probe of the thermometer into the thickest area without touching bone.

3. List the dry-heat methods often used for cooking poultry. roasting, broiling, grilling, frying, oven-frying

   List the moist-heat methods often used for cooking poultry. braising, stewing

4. What does trussing a bird accomplish?
   Trussing prevents the wing and leg tips from overbrowning. It also makes the bird easier to handle and more attractive to serve.

5. If a bird is to be stuffed, when should this be done? Why?
   The bird should be stuffed immediately before it is put into the oven. The bird should not be stuffed until this time to prevent growth of harmful bacteria that can cause foodborne illness.

6. What temperature should stuffing packed into the cavity of a bird reach? at least 165°F (74°C)

7. Why should roasted poultry stand 10 to 15 minutes before it is carved? It will be easier to carve.

8. How can you prevent the breast of a large bird from overbrowning during roasting?
   Make a tent out of aluminum foil. Cover the breast with the foil when the bird is about half cooked.

9. How do cooking bags shorten cooking time? Cooking bags use steam to help cook the bird.

10. When should you thaw frozen poultry? before cooking

(Continued)

11. How can frozen poultry be thawed quickly? _______________________________
    Frozen poultry can be wrapped in a tightly closed plastic bag and placed in a sink full of cold water.
    The water should be changed about every 30 minutes until the bird is defrosted.

12. How far from the heat source should poultry be broiled? 4 to 5 inches

13. How long will it take chicken to broil? about 40 minutes

14. What type of heat should be used when grilling poultry? _______________________________
    Grill poultry with bones using *indirect* heat. Grill boneless poultry pieces over *direct* heat.

15. What are the advantages of partially cooking poultry in a microwave oven before grilling?
    Partially cooking poultry in a microwave oven before grilling shortens grilling time. Partial cooking
    also ensures grilled poultry is thoroughly cooked.

16. How is poultry prepared for frying? _______________________________
    Pieces are rolled in flour, egg, and bread crumbs or dipped in a batter.

17. How deep should the fat be for frying chicken? about ½ inch (1.3 cm)

18. What is another name for oven-frying? baking

19. How can a crisp golden crust be promoted on oven-fried chicken? _______________________________
    Brushing chicken lightly with melted margarine will produce a crisp golden crust.

20. How can you help braised poultry develop a crisp crust? _______________________________
    Uncover the pan for the last 10 minutes of cooking.

21. What ingredients can be added to flavor poultry during stewing? carrots, celery, seasonings

22. How might stewed poultry be used? _______________________________
    Stewed poultry can easily be removed from the bone and used in soups and casseroles.

23. List three benefits of using a microwave oven for preparing poultry. (List three:) Poultry can be
    defrosted quickly in a microwave oven. Poultry can be partially cooked before being prepared by
    another method. Poultry comes out tender and juicy. Poultry cooked in a microwave oven generally
    cooks in much less time than poultry cooked in a conventional oven.

24. How should drumsticks be arranged to ensure even cooking in a microwave oven? _______________________________
    Arrange drumsticks like the spokes of a wheel with the bony portions toward the center and the
    meaty ends toward the outside.

Fish and Shellfish

Nutrition Comparison

Activity A   **Name** _______________________________________

Chapter 20   **Date** ___________________________ **Period** ___________

Compare the nutrition information for the broiled beef top loin steak and the broiled Atlantic salmon to answer the questions that follow. Write your answers in the space provided.

Broiled Beef Top Loin Steak			**Broiled Atlantic Salmon**		
Serving size	1 steak (85 g/3 oz.)		Serving size	1 fillet (85 g/3 oz.)	
Servings per container	4		Servings per container	4	
Calories	224		Calories	174	
Calories from fat	126		Calories from fat	99	
	% daily value			% daily value	
Total fat 14 g	22%		Total fat 11 g	16%	
Saturated fat 6 g	30%		Saturated fat 2 g	11%	
Trans fat 0 g			Trans fat 0 g		
Polyunsaturated fat 1 g			Polyunsaturated fat 4 g		
Monounsaturated fat 6 g			Monounsaturated fat 4 g		
Cholesterol 82 mg	27%		Cholesterol 54 mg	18%	
Sodium 46 mg	2%		Sodium 52 mg	2%	
Total Carbohydrate 0 g			Total Carbohydrate 0 g		
Dietary fiber 0 g			Dietary fiber 0 g		
Sugars 0 g			Sugars 0 g		
Protein 22 g			Protein 19 g		
Vitamin A 0%	Niacin	30%	Vitamin A 1%	Niacin	34%
Vitamin C 0%	Vitamin B_6	24%	Vitamin C 5%	Vitamin B_6	28%
Calcium 2%	Vitamin B_{12}	22%	Calcium 1%	Vitamin B_{12}	40%
Iron 8%	Phosphorus	17%	Iron 2%	Phosphorus	21%
Thiamin 4%	Zinc	27%	Thiamin 19%	Zinc	2%

1. What is the recommendation for including seafood in the diet?______________________
   It is recommended that at least 8 ounce-equivalents per week come from a variety of seafood.

2. How many more calories are provided by a serving of steak than by a serving of salmon? _49_____

3. In terms of percent Daily Value, how much less saturated fat is provided by a serving of salmon? 19%

4. What types of fats should make up the bulk of fats in the diet? ____________________
   Mono- and polyunsaturated fats should make up the bulk of fats in the diet.

5. Which food is lower in cholesterol? salmon ___________________________

6. Which food is the better source of iron? beef top loin steak ___________

7. For which vitamin(s) is the salmon a high source? niacin, vitamin B_6, vitamin B_{12}

8. For which mineral(s) is the beef a high source? zinc _______________________

Choosing Seafood

Name ___________________________

Date ___________________ Period ___________

Match the following descriptions with the terms they describe. Place the correct letters in the corresponding blanks to the left of the numbers.

__E__	1. Fish that have fins and backbones.	A.	crustacean
__J__	2. Fish that have shells instead of backbones.	B.	drawn fish
__H__	3. Fish that have very little fat in their flesh.	C.	dressed fish
__D__	4. Fish having flesh that is fattier than the flesh of lean fish.	D.	fat fish
__B__	5. Fish that has the entrails (insides) removed.	E.	finfish
__C__	6. Fish that has the entrails (insides), head, fins, and scales removed.	F.	fish fillet
__G__	7. Cross-sectional slice taken from a dressed fish.	G.	fish steak
__F__	8. The side of a fish cut lengthwise away from the backbone.	H.	lean fish
__A__	9. Shellfish with a segmented body that is covered by a crustlike shell.	I.	mollusk
__I__	10. Shellfish that has a soft body fully or partially covered by a hard shell.	J.	shellfish
		K.	whole (round) fish

Identify each of the following water animals by the group to which it belongs. Write *L* in the blank if the animal is a lean fish. Write *F* in the blank if the animal is a fat fish. Write *C* in the blank if the animal is a crustacean. Write *M* in the blank if the animal is a mollusk.

__M__	11. clams		__M__	17. oysters
__L__	12. cod		__F__	18. salmon
__C__	13. crabs		__M__	19. scallops
__L__	14. haddock		__C__	20. shrimp
__C__	15. lobster		__L__	21. swordfish
__F__	16. mackerel		__F__	22. trout

23. What is one guideline for buying fresh finfish? (Answers will vary.)

____

24. What is one guideline for buying fresh shellfish? (Answers will vary.)

____

25. What is one guideline for buying frozen or canned seafood? (Answers will vary.)

____

26. What is one guideline for storing seafood? (Answers will vary.)

____

Cooking Finfish

Activity C Name __________________________

Chapter 20 Date __________________________ Period __________

Read the definitions and look at the scrambled letters. Then write the correct terms in the blanks.

1. Cooking in a simmering liquid. GIPHANOC P O A C H I N G

2. Cooking steaks, fillets, or dressed fish under a direct heat source until the fish flakes easily with a fork. LOIBRING B R O I L I N G

3. Cooking steaks, fillets, or dressed fish in the oven. GABNIK B A K I N G

4. Cooking fish on a rack over simmering liquid in a tightly covered pan. MEATSING S T E A M I N G

5. Coating fish with crumbs or batter and then cooking it in fat. YIFRNG F R Y I N G

6. Cooking steaks or fillets directly over hot coals. IIGLGNRL G R I L L I N G

7. Give two tips for preparing seafood that can help you avoid foodborne illness.

   (Answers will vary.)

8. Describe the texture and appearance of finfish cooked to the proper degree of doneness.

   The flesh will be firm and will flake easily with a fork. It will have lost its translucent appearance and will look opaque.

9. Which of the cooking methods described above are recommended for cooking fat fish?

   Broiling, baking, and grilling are recommended methods for cooking fat fish.

10. Which of the cooking methods described above are recommended for cooking lean fish?

    Frying, poaching, and steaming are recommended methods for cooking lean fish.

11. What general guide can be used to time fish cooked by a variety of cooking methods?

    Fish, including stuffed and rolled fish, is measured at its thickest point. It should be cooked about 10 minutes for every inch (2.5 cm) of thickness.

    To what cooking method does this guide not apply?

    This guide does not apply when deep-frying fish.

12. In the space provided, plan a dinner menu that includes a finfish entree.

    (Answers will vary.)

The Fish Market

Name ____

Date _______________________________   Period ____________

Presume you work behind the counter at *Nielsen's Fish Market*. Describe how you would respond to the following questions from some of your regular customers. Write your responses in the space provided.

1. Mrs. Blankenburg is trying to lose weight. She wants to know if eating more fish could help her achieve her goal.

   (Answers will vary.)

   ____

   ____

   ____

2. Mrs. Min is pregnant. She is very concerned about eating a healthful diet that will provide all the nutrients her developing baby needs. She wants to know what nutrients fish will contribute to her diet.

   (Answers will vary.)

   ____

   ____

   ____

3. Mr. Shackelford notices Nielsen's sells only Grade A fish. He says he knows meats are graded by the USDA, but he wants to know who grades fish. He also wants to know what characteristics qualify for a Grade A rating.

   (Answers will vary.)

   ____

   ____

   ____

4. Miss Shelby notices the whole trout in your case. She wants to know if the bulging eyes and red gills indicate the fish may be spoiled.

   (Answers will vary.)

   ____

   ____

   ____

5. Mr. Perry complains your prices are too high. His daughter lives on the coast, and swordfish is much cheaper there. He also wants to avoid paying for a lot of waste.

   (Answers will vary.)

   ____

   ____

   ____

(Continued)

6. Mr. Reed tells you his wife usually does the shopping, but she is out of town. He wants to know how he should store the fresh salmon he is buying. He also wants to know how long it will keep.

   (Answers will vary.)

7. Mrs. Johnson tells you she is afraid of eating undercooked fish. However, the cod she cooked last week came out tough and dry. She wants to know how to tell when fish is properly cooked. She also wants to know how to keep it moist and tender.

   (Answers will vary.)

8. Mr. Ramirez says he always buys halibut and he always steams it. Today he is in the mood for something different. He wants to try catfish, but he is not sure how to cook it.

   (Answers will vary.)

9. Mrs. Petrovski has a busy schedule and is always looking for ways to streamline her meal preparation. She wants to know how much cooking time to allow for the salmon baked in dill sauce she plans to make for dinner this evening.

   (Answers will vary.)

10. Mr. Clark wants to buy and freeze several pounds of the haddock that is on sale this week. He wants to know how to cook frozen fish.

   (Answers will vary.)

Investigating Shellfish

Activity E   Name ____

Chapter 20   Date _______________________   Period ___________

Use Internet and library resources, supermarket research, and the form below to write a brief report about one type of shellfish.

Type of shellfish: _(Answers will vary.)_______________

Parts of the body eaten as food: _(Answers will vary.)______

____

Varieties eaten as food: _(Answers will vary.)__________

____

____

Waters where they are commonly found: ___________
_(Answers will vary.)______________________________

How they are caught: _(Answers will vary.)___________

____

How they are prepared for market:
_(Answers will vary.)______________________________

Market forms: _(Answers will vary.)_________________

Market price range: _(Answers will vary.)____________

How they are commonly cooked: _(Answers will vary.)___

____

Recipe calling for this type of shellfish: _(Answers will vary.)___

Ingredients: _(Answers will vary.)__________________

____

____

Directions: _(Answers will vary.)__________________

____

____

Serves: _(Answers will vary.)____

Salads, Casseroles, and Soups

Salads

Activity A　　　　**Name** ______________________________

Chapter 21　　　　**Date** _______________________　**Period** ___________

Complete the following exercises about salads. Write your responses in the space provided.

1. Explain how to prepare fresh produce for use in a salad. ______________________________
   Wash under clean running water. Trim any bruised or inedible spots. Avoid soaking. Dry gently.

2. Why should salad greens be torn instead of cut with a knife? ______________________________
   Cutting salad greens with a knife can cause bruising.

Match each salad dressing to its description by placing the correct letter in the space provided.

__B__　3. A dressing that is a temporary emulsion made by combining oil,
　　　　　 vinegar, and seasonings.

__C__　4. A dressing containing egg yolks as an emulsifying agent.

__A__　5. A dressing that is a permanent emulsion thickened with a food
　　　　　 starch.

A. cooked salad dressing
B. French dressing
C. mayonnaise
D. Thousand Island dressing

6. Give a specific example of each of the following types of salads.

   Protein salad: _(Answers will vary.)_________________________

   Pasta salad: _(Answers will vary.)_________________________

   Vegetable salad: _(Answers will vary.)_________________________

   Fruit salad: _(Answers will vary.)_________________________

   Gelatin salad: _(Answers will vary.)_________________________

7. Create a salad. List the ingredients to be included in the salad. Then draw a sketch of the salad. Label
   the base, body, dressing, and garnish parts of the salad.

   Ingredients: _(Answers will vary.)_____________　　　Sketch:

   ____

   ____

   ____

   ____

   ____

Casserole Preparation Guide

Activity B   Name ____

Chapter 21   Date _______________________   Period ____________

List five items in each of the casserole ingredient categories below. Then answer the questions that follow to provide tips on putting a casserole together.   (Chart answers will vary.)

Protein Foods	Vegetables
A.	A.
B.	B.
C.	C.
D.	D.
E.	E.
Starchy Foods	**Sauces**
A.	A.
B.	B.
C.	C.
D.	D.
E.	E.
Extras	**Toppings**
A.	A.
B.	B.
C.	C.
D.	D.
E.	E.

1. How can casseroles help stretch food dollars? Casseroles can stretch food dollars by using starchy foods and vegetables to extend more costly protein ingredients.

2. How can casseroles help people emphasize plant foods in their diets? Casseroles often include a variety of vegetables and grains and only a small amount of meat. Many casseroles can be made without meat.

3. Give a suggestion for reducing the fat and sodium in a casserole recipe. Use reduced-fat mayonnaise or low-sodium condensed soup in place of traditional ingredients.

4. How can cleanup of baked casseroles be made easier? Cleanup is easier by putting casseroles into a greased dish.

5. How can the topping on a casserole be kept from getting too dark? Loosely place a piece of aluminum foil over the top of the casserole.

Stock Soups

Name ____

Date ___________________________ Period ____________

Match the following descriptions with the appropriate terms by placing the correct letter in the blank provided to the left of each number.

___E___ 1. The stock resulting when poultry, fish, or unbrowned meat is cooked in a liquid.

___B___ 2. The stock resulting when browned meat is cooked in a liquid.

___F___ 3. A process done to separate broth from solid materials.

___C___ 4. The stock that results when slightly beaten egg white and a few pieces of eggshell are added to a boiling broth.

___A___ 5. A clear broth made from stock.

___D___ 6. A clear, rich-flavored soup made from stock.

A. bouillon
B. brown stock
C. clarified stock
D. consommé
E. light stock
F. straining
G. unbrowned stock

The steps required for preparing bouillon are listed below. Place the numbers 1 through 10 in the blanks to reorganize the steps in the correct order.

___6___ 7. Fat is removed from the surface of the stock.

___9___ 8. The clarified stock is strained to remove the egg, solid materials, and eggshell.

___3___ 9. The ingredients are placed in a large pan and covered with water.

___4___ 10. The pan is covered with a tightly fitted lid and the ingredients are simmered for several hours.

___1___ 11. The meat and vegetables to be used in the stock are cut into small pieces.

___10___ 12. The strained, clarified stock is reduced in volume by further cooking.

___7___ 13. The stock is strained to separate the solid materials from the broth.

___5___ 14. Foam is skimmed from the surface of the stock.

___8___ 15. The stock is clarified.

___2___ 16. The meat is browned.

Foods like soups, salads, and casseroles include foods from more than one MyPlate food group. Identify the amounts from each food group that would be provided by a serving of the following recipe.

Chicken Noodle Soup

Makes 12 servings

12	cups low-sodium chicken broth	1	cup sliced celery
1	bay leaf	1	cup sliced carrots
½	teaspoon sage	1	cup chopped mushrooms
½	teaspoon thyme	1	cup chopped onion
1¾	teaspoons salt	6	cups cooked wide egg noodles
	Fresh ground pepper	8	small boneless, skinless chicken breast halves, cooked and diced

17. Fruit group: ___0___ cups

18. Vegetable group: ___⅓___ cups

19. Grains group: ___1___ oz. eq.

20. Protein foods group: ___2___ oz. eq.

21. Dairy group: ___0___ cups

Herbs, Spices, and Blends

Activity D   Name ____

Chapter 21   Date ___________________________   Period ____________

List the seasonings you have in your foods laboratory. Check the appropriate column to indicate whether each is an herb, a spice, or a blend. Identify the type(s) of food(s) in which each seasoning is used. Then complete the items at the bottom of the page. (Chart answers will vary.)

Seasoning	Type (✓)			Used to Flavor
	Herb	**Spice**	**Blend**	

1. Explain how herbs, spices, and blends differ.

   Herbs are the leaves of plants usually grown in temperate climates. Spices are the dried roots, stems, and seeds of plants grown mainly in the tropics. Blends are combinations of herbs and spices.

2. Describe how to store herbs, spices, and blends properly.

   Always store herbs, spices, and blends in a cool, dry place away from light. Keep the containers tightly closed.

Breads

Functions of Ingredients

Activity A **Name** ____

Chapter 22 **Date** _____________________________ **Period** _____________

The principle ingredients used in baked products are pictured in the following. In the space provided, list at least one function of each of these ingredients in baked products.

A. _(Answers will vary. See text page 388.)_

B. _(Answers will vary. See text pages 388–389.)_

C. _(Answers will vary. See text pages 388–389.)_

D. _(Answers will vary. See text page 395)_

E. _(Answers will vary. See text page 390.)_

F. _(Answers will vary. See text page 389.)_

G. _(Answers will vary. See text page 391.)_

H. _(Answers will vary. See text page 389.)_

I. _(Answers will vary. See text page 390.)_

Adjusting Recipes

Name _______________________________

Date _____________________ Period ___________

Rewrite the ingredient list for the recipe below to reflect minimum ingredient proportions. Write your response in the space provided.

<table>
<tr><td colspan="2">Old-Fashioned Biscuits
(Makes 12 biscuits)</td><td colspan="2">Healthy Biscuits
(Makes 12 biscuits)</td></tr>
<tr><td>2 cups all-purpose flour</td><td></td><td>1 cup all-purpose flour</td></tr>
<tr><td>2 teaspoons sugar</td><td></td><td>1 cup whole-wheat flour (omit sugar)</td></tr>
<tr><td>1 tablespoon baking powder</td><td></td><td>2¾ teaspoons baking powder</td></tr>
<tr><td>1 teaspoon salt</td><td></td><td>½ teaspoon salt</td></tr>
<tr><td>⅓ cup shortening</td><td></td><td>¼ cup shortening</td></tr>
<tr><td>¾ cup milk</td><td></td><td>¾ cup fat-free milk</td></tr>
</table>

Use the following information to calculate the changes in nutritional value that will result from making these adjustments to the recipe:

- Sugar provides 15 calories per teaspoon.
- Baking powder provides 390 mg of sodium per teaspoon.
- Salt provides 2,000 mg of sodium per teaspoon.
- Shortening provides 115 calories and 13 g of fat per tablespoon.
- Fat-free milk provides 65 fewer calories and 8 g less fat per cup than whole milk.

1. Total calorie savings _279 calories_

2. Calorie savings per biscuit _23 calories_

3. Total fat savings _23 grams of fat_

4. Fat savings per biscuit _2 grams of fat_

5. Total sodium savings _1, 293 milligrams of sodium_

6. Sodium savings per biscuit _100 milligrams of sodium_

7. Total fiber increase _10 grams of fiber_

8. Fiber increase per biscuit _1 gram of fiber_

9. Based on the changes that resulted from adjusting the above recipe, would you be inclined to adjust other recipes you prepare? Explain why or why not. _______________________

   (Answers will vary.)

Characteristics of Quick Breads

Activity C   **Name** _______________________________________

Chapter 22   **Date** ____________________________ **Period** _____________

Answer the following questions about the characteristics of quick breads in the space provided.

1. What role does gluten play in the preparation of quick breads? _______________________
   Gluten is a protein that gives strength and elasticity to batters and doughs and structure to baked
   products. It also holds the leavening gases, which make quick breads rise.

2. How is gluten formed? ____
   Gluten is created by the proteins *gliadin* and *glutenin*, which are found in wheat flour. When flour is
   combined with liquid and the mixture is stirred or kneaded, the gliadin and glutenin form gluten.

3. What are two differences between rolled biscuits and dropped biscuits? (List two:) Dropped biscuits
   have a higher proportion of liquid than rolled biscuits. Rolled biscuits are cut with a biscuit cutter;
   dropped biscuits are dropped from a spoon. Rolled biscuits are baked on an ungreased baking sheet;
   dropped biscuits are baked on a greased baking sheet.

4. Describe the characteristics of a high-quality rolled biscuit. A high-quality rolled biscuit has an even
   shape with a smooth, level top and straight sides. The crust is an even brown. The interior is white to
   creamy white. The crumb is moist and fluffy and peels off in layers.

5. Read the characteristics below. Write *O* in the blank if the characteristic describes an overmixed
   muffin. Write *U* in the blank if the characteristic describes an undermixed muffin. Write *H* in the blank
   if the characteristic describes a high-quality muffin.

__U__	A. coarse crumb		__H__	F. symmetrical top that looks rough
__U__	B. flat top		__H__	G. tender, light crumb
__U__	C. low volume		__H__	H. thin, evenly browned crust
__O__	D. pale, slick crust		__O__	I. tunnels
__O__	E. peaked top		__H__	J. uniform texture

6. Why is the oven temperature for popovers changed partway through the baking period? A hot oven is
   used for the first part of the baking period to allow steam to expand the walls of the popovers. A lower
   temperature is used during the second part of the baking period to prevent overbrowning.

7. What happens to a popover that has not been baked long enough? ____________________
   A popover that has not been baked long enough will collapse when it is taken from the oven. The
   exterior will be soft instead of crisp, and the interior will be doughy.

8. What can happen to cream puffs if the oven door is opened during baking? _______________
   If the cream puffs have not set, the steam can condense and cause them to collapse.

9. What occasionally causes cream puffs to ooze fat during baking? _____________________
   The evaporation of too much liquid occasionally causes cream puffs to ooze fat during baking. This
   might occur when the water and fat are heated together or when the puff paste is cooked.

10. How should freshly baked items be stored? _______________________________________
    Store freshly baked items at room temperature or in the freezer, tightly wrapped.

Yeast Breads

Complete the following exercises dealing with yeast breads. Write your responses in the space provided.

1. How does bread flour differ from all-purpose flour and why is it recommended when preparing breads in a bread machine?

    Bread flour contains larger amounts of gliadin and glutenin than all-purpose flour, so it produces the strongest and most elastic gluten. It is recommended when making bread in a bread machine because the actions of a bread machine require stronger gluten.

2. What effect does milk have when used as the liquid in a yeast bread recipe?

    Milk produces a softer crust and helps breads stay fresh longer than water does.

3. How does fast-rising yeast differ from active dry yeast? The granules of fast-rising yeast are smaller than those of active dry yeast, which allows them to act more quickly.

Match the following mixing methods for yeast breads with their descriptions.

  E   4. Doughs prepared by this method are allowed to rise twice.   A. batter method

  D   5. This method requires the use of fast-rising yeast.   B. biscuit method

  C   6. In this method, using an electric mixer helps develop gluten and shorten the kneading time.   C. mixer method

                            D. one-rise method

  A   7. Vigorous stirring, rather than kneading, helps develop the gluten in this method.   E. traditional method

8. Why is yeast bread kneaded? ____

    Bread is kneaded to develop gluten.

9. How can you tell whether yeast dough has doubled in volume during fermentation? ____________

    Gently push two fingers into the dough. If an indentation remains, the dough has doubled in volume.

10. Why does yeast dough need to be punched? _____________________________________

    Yeast dough needs to be punched to release some of the carbon dioxide.

11. Characteristics of yeast breads are listed below. Check those that are signs of a high-quality loaf of yeast bread.

     ✓ A. large volume   ✓ F. fine, uniform texture

         B. small volume   G. crumbly

     ✓ C. smooth, rounded top   ✓ H. tender, elastic crumb

         D. sunken top with overhanging sides   I. contains large, overexpanded cells

         E. coarse texture   J. compact texture

12. Describe two time-saving techniques for preparing yeast breads. ______________________

    (Describe two. Answers will vary.)

    ____

    ____

Cakes, Cookies, Pies, and Candies

Kinds of Cakes

Activity A Name ____

Chapter 23 Date ____________________ Period ____________

Complete the following exercises about cakes. Write your responses in the space provided.

1. Check all the following characteristics that apply to shortened cakes.

   ✓ A. They contain fat.

   ___ B. They contain no fat.

   ✓ C. Butter cake is an example of a shortened cake.

   ___ D. A sponge cake is an example of a shortened cake.

   ✓ E. They usually contain leavening agents.

   ✓ F. They are tender, moist, and velvety.

2. How do pound cakes differ from other shortened cakes? ________________________
   Pound cakes contain no chemical leavening agents. They are more compact than other shortened cakes, and they have a closer grain.

3. Check all the following characteristics that apply to unshortened cakes.

   ✓ A. They are sometimes called foam cakes.

   ✓ B. They contain no fat.

   ✓ C. Angel food cake is an example of an unshortened cake.

   ___ D. Chocolate cakes are unshortened cakes.

   ✓ E. They are leavened by air and steam.

4. How do sponge cakes differ from other unshortened cakes? ________________________
   Sponge cakes contain the whole egg rather than just the egg white.

5. Check all the following characteristics that apply to chiffon cakes.

   ✓ A. They contain fat.

   ✓ B. They contain beaten egg whites.

   ✓ C. They are a cross between shortened and unshortened cakes.

   ___ D. They contain no eggs or fat.

Match each of the basic ingredients to the fuction it performs in cakes by placing the correct letter in the corresponding blank.

H	6. Gives sweetness, tenderizes the gluten, and improves the texture.	A. cream of tartar
D	7. Gives structure to a cake.	B. egg
E	8. Causes a cake to rise.	C. fat
C	9. Tenderizes the gluten.	D. flour
A	10. Used in angel food and sponge cakes to make the grain finer and to stabilize the egg white proteins.	E. leavening agent
		F. liquid
G or I	11. Provides flavoring.	G. salt
B	12. Improves the flavor and color and helps leaven some cakes.	H. sugar
F	13. Provides moisture and helps blend ingredients.	I. vanilla extract

Preparing Cakes

Activity B   **Name** _______________________________________

Chapter 23   **Date** _____________________   **Period** ____________

The statements that follow describe preparation principles and techniques used in preparing cakes. In the space provided, give a reason for each principle or step.

Principles of Preparation

1. Measure the flour accurately. A cake made with too much flour is compact and dry. A cake made with too little four is coarse, and it may fall.

2. Avoid overmixing the ingredients. Overmixing causes the gluten to overdevelop and the cake will be tough.

3. Bake the batter in pans of the correct size. If the pans are too small, the batter will overflow. If the pans are too large, the cake will be too flat and may be dry.

4. Do not grease pans for unshortened cakes. Angel food and sponge cake batters must cling to the sides of the pan during baking.

5. Bake the cake just until it tests done. Cakes baked too long may be dry.

Baking Shortened Cakes

6. Pans should not touch each other or the oven while baking. This allows the heat to circulate freely and prevents hot spots and uneven baking.

7. Insert a wooden toothpick into the center of the cake or lightly touch the center of the cake with your fingertip. If the toothpick comes out clean or the cake springs back when touched, the cake is done.

8. Allow the cake to cool in the pan for about 10 minutes. This makes it easier to remove the cake from the pan.

9. Run the tip of a metal spatula around the sides of the baked cake. This loosens the cake before removing it from the pan.

Preparing Unshortened Cakes

10. Ingredients should be at room temperature. This allows the egg whites to achieve maximum volume when they are beaten.

11. After pouring batter into the pan, run a spatula through the batter. This releases large air bubbles and seals the batter against the sides of the pan.

12. Gently touch the cracks that form in the top of the cake. If the cracks feel dry and no imprint remains, the cake is done.

13. When the cake is done, place the cake upside down over the neck of a bottle. This prevents loss of volume during cooling.

Cookies

Name ______________________________

Date ________________________ Period ____________

Match the following descriptions with the kinds of cookies they describe. Place the letter of the correct answer in the space provided to the left of each number.

___F___ 1. A stiff dough rolled to a thickness of 1/8 to 1/4 inch and cut with a cookie cutter.

___B___ 2. A soft dough pushed from a spoon onto a cookie sheet.

___A___ 3. A soft dough spread evenly in a jelly roll pan or square pan.

___E___ 4. A stiff dough formed into a long roll that is cut into thin slices.

___D___ 5. A very rich, stiff dough that is packed into a utensil and pushed through perforated disks onto a cookie sheet.

___C___ 6. A stiff dough broken into small pieces and shaped with the fingers.

A. bar cookies
B. drop cookies
C. molded cookies
D. pressed cookies
E. refrigerator cookies
F. rolled cookies
G. shaped cookies

Read the following statements about cookies. Circle *T* if the statement is true. Circle *F* if the statement is false.

(T) F   7. Although the ingredients used to make different kinds of cookies are similar, the doughs differ in consistency.

T (F)   8. Drop cookies do not spread as much as rolled cookies during baking.

(T) F   9. Refrigerator cookies contain a high proportion of fat.

T (F) 10. Chocolate chip cookies are popular molded cookies.

(T) F 11. Most cookies contain more fat and sugar and less liquid than cakes.

T (F) 12. The conventional mixing method used for shortened cakes is used to mix all types of cookies.

(T) F 13. Cookie sheets should not have high sides, or cookies will bake unevenly.

T (F) 14. Cookies baked on bright, shiny cookie sheets will have dark bottoms.

T (F) 15. Cookie sheets should be hot when cookies are placed on them for baking.

T (F) 16. Cookie sheets should touch the sides of the oven when cookies are baking.

T (F) 17. Crisp cookies should be stored in a container with a tight-fitting cover.

(T) F 18. Many cookies freeze well both in dough form and after baking.

(T) F 19. Frozen dough for drop cookies needs to be thawed before it is dropped and baked.

T (F) 20. Crisp cookies that have become soft can be made crisp again by placing a piece of bread in the cookie container.

Pie Filling

Name _______________________________

Date _____________________ Period ____________

Supply the requested information about different kinds of pies. Write your responses in the space provided in the diagram.

1. Describe a typical fruit pie.
A fruit pie is typically a two-crust pie with a filling made from canned, frozen, dried, or fresh fruit or commercially prepared pie filling.

2. Describe a typical cream pie.
A cream pie is typically a one-crust pie with a filling made from a cornstarch-thickened pudding mixture.

3. Describe a typical custard pie.
A custard pie is typically a one-crust pie filled with custard made from milk, eggs, and sugar.

4. Describe a typical chiffon pie.
A chiffon pie is typically a one-crust pie filled with a light, airy mixture containing gelatin and cooked beaten egg whites.

5. Describe the characteristics of a high-quality pie.
A high-quality pie has a tender, flaky, crisp crust. It should be evenly browned and the filling should have a pleasing flavor and texture.

6. Describe your favorite kind of pie.
(Answers will vary.)

Pastry Preparation

Activity E   Name ______________________________________

Chapter 23   Date ____________________________   Period ____________

Place a check mark next to the best response for each item.

1. What are the four basic ingredients used to make pastry?

   _____ A. Flour, eggs, leavening, liquid.   _____ C. Fruit filling, meringue, custard, gelatin.

   ✔ B. Flour, fat, water, salt.   _____ D. Milk, eggs, sugar, flour.

2. What is the function of flour in pastry?

   _____ A Contributes to flakiness.   _____ C. Produces steam.

   _____ B. Contributes flavor.   ✔ D. Provides structure.

3. What is the function of salt in pastry?

   ✔ A. Contributes flavor.   _____ C. Promotes gluten development.

   _____ B. Inhibits gluten development.   _____ D. Provides structure.

4. How does fat perform in pastry?

   _____ A. It creates a framework that traps air.   ✔ C. It prevents too much water from coming in contact with the flour.

   _____ B. It moistens the flour so gluten will develop.   _____ D. It produces steam needed for flakiness.

5. Which of the following can make pastry tough?

   _____ A. Too little handling.   _____ C. Too little flour.

   _____ B. Too much fat.   ✔ D. Too much liquid.

6. Which of the following is a guideline for producing pastry that is tender and flaky?

   ✔ A. Handle pastry as little as possible.   _____ C. Stretch the pastry when fitting it into the pie plate.

   _____ B. Knead the pastry gently.   _____ D. Use the rolling pin vigorously when rolling pastry.

7. The most common method for mixing pastry is the ______.

   ✔ A. biscuit method   _____ C. muffin method

   _____ B. conventional method   _____ D. pie method

8. When making a one-crust pie that will be filled after baking, ______.

   _____ A. do not prick the bottom or sides of the piecrust before baking it   ✔ C. prick the bottom and sides of the piecrust before baking it

   _____ B. make several small slits in the piecrust before baking it   _____ D. thoroughly chill the piecrust before filling it

          Chapter 23   Cakes, Cookies, Pies, and Candies

Candy

Name ______________________________

Date ______________________ **Period** ___________

Read the clues that follow. Write *C* in the blank if the clue describes crystalline candy. Write *NC* in the blank if the clue describes noncrystalline candy. If the clue describes both types of candy, write *B* in the blank.

__C__ 1. Fudge is an example.

__NC__ 2. Caramels are an example.

__NC__ 3. Peanut brittle is an example.

__C__ 4. Divinity is an example.

__NC__ 5. Toffee is an example.

__C__ 6. Fondant is an example.

__B__ 7. A sugar syrup is used.

__C__ 8. The sugar syrup is heated to a specific temperature, cooled to a specific temperature, and beaten vigorously.

__NC__ 9. The sugar syrup is heated to a very high temperature.

__NC__ 10. Substances such as corn syrup, milk, cream, or butter are added to interfere with crystallization.

__B__ 11. A candy thermometer is used for accuracy.

__B__ 12. The use of a heavy saucepan or iron skillet is recommended.

__B__ 13. For best results, follow the recipe exactly.

__C__ 14. The sugar syrup forms small, fine crystals.

__NC__ 15. The sugar syrup does not form crystals.

16. What is sugar syrup and what does it have to do with candy making? Sugar syrup is a heated mixture of sugar and liquid that is the basis of all cooked candies.

17. Describe high-quality fudge. High-quality fudge tastes smooth and creamy because it contains small sugar crystals. It has a deep brown color and a satiny sheen.

18. Describe high-quality peanut brittle. High-quality peanut brittle has a golden color and looks foamy.

19. What are three ways of using chocolate to make simple candies? Melted chocolate can be poured into molds; used to make clusters of raisins, nuts, or coconut; and used to dip fondant or caramels.

20. How should chocolate be prepared for melting? Chop bars into small pieces or use chocolate chips.

21. What is cocoa butter and what does it have to do with chocolate? Cocoa butter is the fat from cacao beans. High cocoa butter content is a sign of quality in chocolate.

22. Why is white chocolate not considered to be true chocolate? It contains no chocolate liquor.

Food and Entertaining

Planning a Social Gathering

Activity A   **Name** ___________________________________

Chapter 24   **Date** _____________________   **Period** ____________

Choose a theme for a social gathering. Complete the following invitation with the date, time, place, and any other information guests will need to know. Then complete the planning activities that follow. Write your responses in the space provided.

You Are Invited To:

What? (Answers will vary.) ___________________________

When? _______________________________________

Where? _______________________________________

R.S.V.P. _______________________________________

What factors will affect the number of people invited to this gathering?

(Answers will vary.) _______________________________________

How many people will be invited? (Answers will vary.) _______________________________

Think about who might be invited to this gathering. What interests do these people share that will help them get to know one another?

(Answers will vary.) _______________________________________

In the space provided, plan a menu of familiar recipes for the event described in the invitation. Be sure to list only items for which all the needed equipment is available.

(Answers will vary.) _______________________   _______________________

_______________________   _______________________

_______________________   _______________________

_______________________   _______________________

Describe how the planned refreshments or meal will be served.

(Answers will vary.) _______________________________________

____

(Continued)

What is the budget for the gathering? $ (Answers will vary.)

How much will be spent for the food items listed in the menu?   – (Answers will vary.)

How much will be left to spend on decorations and entertainment? $ (Answers will vary.)

Put a star beside each of the items in the menu on the previous page that can be prepared in advance. In the following table, plan a time schedule for preparing the remaining menu items on the day of the event.

Time	Tasks

What, if any, decorating will be done for this event?

(Answers will vary.)

____

How will guests dress for this event?

(Answers will vary.)

____

Make a list of what needs to be done, besides preparing food, to get ready for this event.

(Answers will vary.)

____

Describe a planned activity that would break the ice and help guests get to know one another.

(Answers will vary.)

____

List three responsibilities of a good guest.

1. (Answers will vary.)

2. (Answers will vary.)

3. (Answers will vary.)

Meal Service

Name ____

Date ________________________________ **Period** _____________

The six major styles of meal service are in the list that follows. Read the meal service descriptions below the list. In the space to the left of each number, write the letter of the meal-service style to which it corresponds. (Some letters will be used more than once.)

A. American or family style service
B. Russian or continental service
C. English service
D. compromise service
E. blue plate service
F. buffet service

___C___ 1. Because this style of service requires a lot of passing, it is best used with small groups.

___F___ 2. A style of meal service in which guests serve themselves from a table that holds serving pieces and tableware.

___A___ 3. Serving dishes are passed around the table, and diners serve themselves.

___B___ 4. Serving dishes are never placed on the table.

___C___ 5. The host fills plates at the table and passes them around the table until each guest has been served.

___B___ 6. This is the most formal style of meal service.

___A___ 7. This is the style of meal service used most often in homes in the United States.

___D___ 8. This is a combination of Russian service and English service.

___E___ 9. Plates are filled in the kitchen, carried into the dining room, and served.

___B___ 10. Guests are served filled plates of food by the waiters.

Read the following statements about waiting on the table. If the statement is true, circle the *T*. If the statement is false, circle the *F*.

(T) F 11. The style of service helps determine the way in which the table is cleared and new courses are served.

T (F) 12. The table is cleared in a clockwise direction.

(T) F 13. The person seated to the right of the host is usually served first.

(T) F 14. When serving, the server should stand at the guest's left side and place the plate with the left hand.

(T) F 15. When clearing a course, the serving dishes should be removed first.

(T) F 16. A small tray should be used to remove items that will not be needed for the next course.

T (F) 17. Water is poured from the left side with the left hand.

T (F) 18. When serving a new course, the first step is to place the needed dinnerware at each cover.

Table Manners

Activity C   Name ____________________________

Chapter 24   Date ____________________   Period ___________

Answer the following questions about situations that require table manners. Write your responses in the space provided to the right of each situation.

1. What should Jacob do with his napkin when he sits down at the table?

   1. Open the napkin to a comfortable size and place it on his lap.

2. The salad has tomatoes on it, and Roland is allergic to tomatoes. What should he do?

   2. Leave the tomatoes on the plate without comment.

3. There are three forks next to Ayanna's plate. How can she know which one to use first?

   3. Eating utensils are used in the order in which they are placed on the table—from the outside toward the plate.

4. Matthew dropped his spoon. What should he do?

   4. He should not use the spoon anymore. Matthew's host should get him another one.

5. The salad dressing Madison would like is across the table. How should she get it?

   5. She should ask for the dressing to be passed.

6. How should Emily eat the bread her host serves with the meal?

   6. Emily should tear the bread into quarters and butter only one quarter at a time.

7. Michael has an olive pit in his mouth. How should he remove it?

   7. Michael should remove the pit from his mouth with his fingers as inconspicuously as possible.

8. Shan's host serves fried chicken at a rather formal meal. How should he eat it?

   8. Shan should use utensils when eating fried chicken at a formal gathering.

9. Hannah starts having a coughing spell in the middle of dinner. What should she do?

   9. Hannah should use her handkerchief, quietly excuse herself, and leave the table.

10. Joshua has just finished eating. What should he do with his flatware?

    10. Joshua should place his knife on the rim of the plate with the sharp edge pointing toward the center and place his fork parallel to the knife.

Outdoor Entertaining

Activity D   **Name** ___________________________________

Chapter 24   **Date** ___________________________   **Period** ___________

Presume you are the recreation services director at *Evergreen Lake Park*, a large facility with a conference center and full-service kitchen. Your many responsibilities include planning seasonal activities that will appeal to members of the community and generate operating funds for the park. Complete the following items to help with your summer event planning.

1. You can offer a *Bicyclist's Box Lunch* for guests riding the multipurpose trail around the lake.

   Plan a menu for the kitchen staff to pack.

   (Answers will vary.)

   Why are these foods good choices for a bicycle picnic?

   (Answers will vary.)

2. You have scheduled weekly cookouts with entertainment on the patio outside the conference center. Check which of the following instructions you will give the staff who will be setting up the grills and cooking.

   _____ A. Place the grills right outside the conference center doors for convenient access to the kitchen.

   ✓ B. Place the grills on the open patio, away from shrubs, furniture, and the conference center.

   ✓ C. Wear tight-fitting clothes and a heavy-duty apron.

   _____ D. Wear loose clothes for comfort and ease of movement.

   _____ E. Keep extra lighter fluid close by in case you need to add more after lighting the coals.

   ✓ F. Never pour lighter fluid over the coals once the fire has started.

   _____ G. Light the charcoal about an hour before you plan to begin cooking.

   ✓ H. Light the charcoal about 30 minutes before you plan to begin cooking.

   ✓ I. Begin cooking when the coals are covered with gray ash.

   _____ J. Begin cooking when the coals are glowing red.

   _____ K. Set out the food for the grill well in advance so you can be sure you have everything you need.

   ✓ L. Keep the food for the grill in coolers until the coals are ready.

3. The conference center already owns large grills to use for summer events. What other grilling equipment will you order for the staff to use at the cookouts?

   tongs, long-handled forks, broad turners, basting brushes, fireproof mitts, heavy-duty foil, food thermometers

Dining Out

Name ___________________________________

Date _______________________ Period ___________

Suppose your boss wants you to put together a local dining guide to assist out-of-town clients. List the name of a restaurant in your area for each of the restaurant types in the following table. Then complete the table with information about the specific restaurants you listed. Consider using the entertainment section of a newspaper or metropolitan magazine to help complete this activity. (Table answers will vary.)

Type of Restaurant	Atmosphere	Menu Items Available	Price Range	Popular Characteristics
Fast-food restaurant				
Cafeteria/ Buffet				
Family restaurant				
Formal restaurant				
Specialty restaurant				

Which of the above restaurants would you recommend to clients? Explain your answer.

(Answers will vary.)

____

____

____

____

Preserving Foods

Microorganisms and Enzymes

Activity A **Name** _______________________________

Chapter 25 **Date** _____________________ **Period** ___________

Read the following phrases. If the phrase describes microorganisms, circle *M*. If the phrase describes enzymes, circle *E*. Then answer the questions that follow. Write your responses in the space provided.

(M) E 1. They include bacteria, mold, and yeast.

M (E) 2. They are complex proteins produced by living cells.

(M) E 3. They are used in making buttermilk and sauerkraut.

(M) E 4. They are used in curing some cheeses such as Roquefort and Camembert.

M (E) 5. They ripen foods.

M (E) 6. They tenderize meats.

M (E) 7. They can cause foods to deteriorate.

(M) E 8. They need food, moisture, and favorable temperatures to grow.

(M) E 9. Their growth is prevented by freezing temperatures.

M (E) 10. Their action is retarded by freezing temperatures.

11. Describe how bacteria, mold, yeast, and enzymes can negatively affect the quality of foods._________
Bacteria can cause foodborne illness and chemical reactions that lead to food spoilage. Mold is a
growth that can appear on foods. Yeast can cause fermentation in preserved food, which results in
spoilage. Enzymes can soften the texture, change the color, and impair the flavor of foods.

12. Describe how freezing temperatures affect microorganisms and enzymes. ___________________
Freezing temperatures prevent microorganisms from growing and retard the action of enzymes.

13. Describe how high temperatures, such as those used in canning, affect microorganisms and enzymes.
High temperatures destroy microorganisms and enzymes.

14. Describe how drying prevents the growth of microorganisms and controls enzyme activity.
Drying removes the moisture needed for microorganism growth. Treatment before drying controls
enzyme activity.

Home Canning

Activity B Name ____

Chapter 25 Date _________________________ Period ______________

Select the answer that *best* completes each of the following statements and write the letter in the blank to the left of each number.

__A__ 1. Most foods are canned at home in ______.
  A. glass jars B. aluminum cans

__B__ 2. A flat metal lid for a home canning jar should be ______.
  A. reused B. used only once

__B__ 3. When canning foods that are processed less than 10 minutes, the canning jars need to be ______.
  A. new B. sterilized

__B__ 4. Packing raw fruits or vegetables into canning jars and covering the food with boiling water, juice, or syrup is called the ______ method.
  A. hot pack B. raw pack

__A__ 5. Pressure canning is used for ______ foods.
  A. low-acid B. high-acid

__B__ 6. In a pressure canner, steam is released through the ______.
  A. pressure gauge B. petcock

__B__ 7. Boiling water canning would be suitable for ______.
  A. green beans B. peaches

__B__ 8. In boiling water canning, processing time begins when ______.
  A. the canner is placed on the heat B. the water comes to a rolling boil

__A__ 9. When canning jars are completely cool, screw bands are ______.
  A. carefully removed B. left on for storage

__A__ 10. Home-canned foods should be stored in a ______ place.
  A. cool, dry, dark B. cool, moist, dark

Read the following statements about checking for spoilage in home-canned foods. If the statement is true, circle *T*. If the statement is false, circle *F*.

(T) F 11. Bulging lids and leaks are signs of broken seals and spoilage.

T (F) 12. If you believe a home-canned food is spoiled, taste it to be certain.

(T) F 13. Botulism is the most dangerous type of foodborne illness.

(T) F 14. Some spoiled foods may look and smell normal.

(T) F 15. If a home-canned food looks spoiled, foams, or has an off odor during heating, destroy it.

Jellied Products Crossword

Activity C

Chapter 25

Name _______________________________________

Date _____________________________ Period ____________

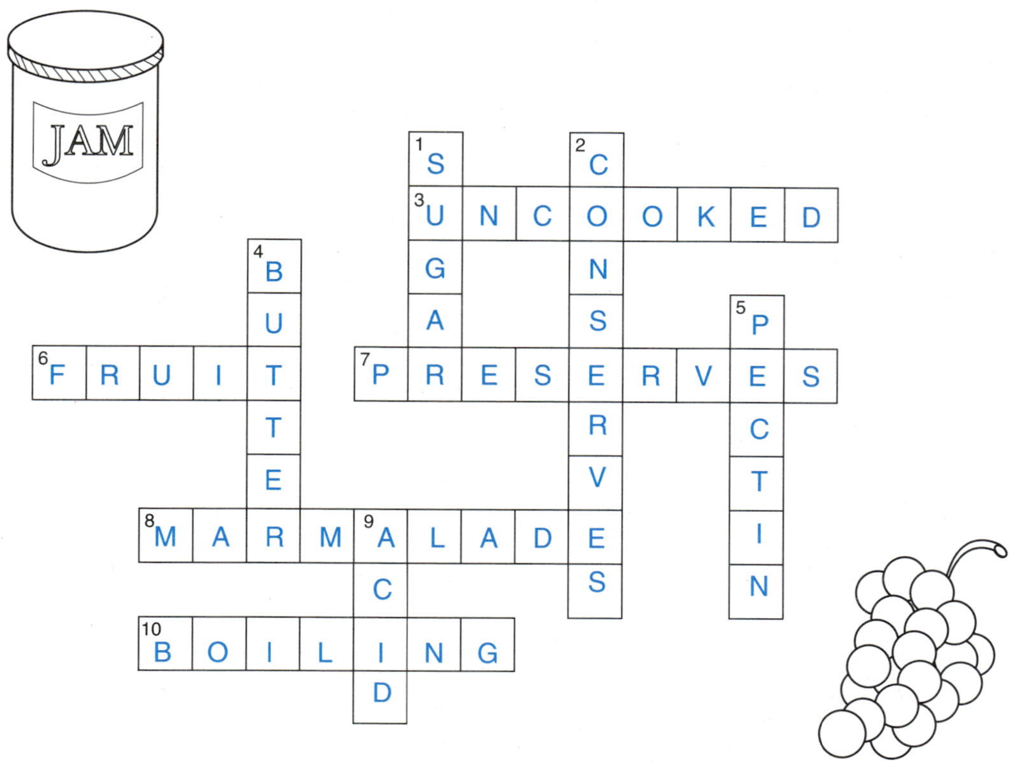

Across

3. _______ jam keeps up to three weeks in the refrigerator, but it spoils quickly at room temperature.
6. _______ is the basic ingredient that gives jellied products their flavors and colors.
7. Slightly jellied products that contain whole or large pieces of fruit in thick syrup are called _______.
8. _______ is a tender jelly often made from citrus fruits.
10. Jellied products must be processed by the _______ water method.

Down

1. _______ helps jelly become firm.
2. Raisins and nuts are sometimes added to _______.
4. Fruit _______ is made from cooked, pureed fruit, but it is not a jellied product.
5. _______ is a carbohydrate found in all fruits that makes fruit juices jell.
9. _______ works along with pectin to make fruit juices jell.

Freezing

Name ___________________________

Date ___________________________   Period ____________

Complete the following statements about freezing food. Then arrange the circled letters to spell a term related to freezing food. Answer the questions that follow.

1. Foods preserved by Q U I C K - F R E E Z I N G are subjected to temperatures between –25°F and –40°F (–32°C and –40°C) for a short time.

2. If food is frozen slowly, large I C E C R Y S T A L S may form and damage the cell structure of the food and change its texture.

3. The main piece of equipment required to freeze food is a properly operating F R E E Z E R.

4. Containers used in freezing must be moisture- and V A P O R -resistant to protect food from exposure to air and loss of moisture.

5. Dry, tough areas that occur where dry air from the freezer comes in contact with food surfaces is called F R E E Z E R B U R N.

6. C O N T A I N E R S made of plastic, glass, aluminum, and plastic-coated paper are suitable for freezer storage.

7. When selecting produce for freezing, choose R I P E, top-quality fruits and young, tender vegetables.

8. Fruits are often treated with A S C O R B I C acid before freezing to preserve color and flavor and add nutritive value.

9. Most vegetables must be B L A N C H E D in boiling water or steam before freezing to inactivate enzymes that can cause spoilage.

10. When packing foods to be frozen, leave 1 inch (2.5 cm) of H E A D S P A C E to allow for expansion.

11. When freezing meats, you may wish to trim large cuts and package them in appropriate S E R V I N G-sized pieces.

12. Thawing fruits in their original covered containers will prevent discoloration caused by exposure to air, which is called E N Z Y M A T I C B R O W N I N G.

Circled letters: I, S, E, O, R, T, P, R, N, E, V, A

Freezing is one method of food P R E S E R V A T I O N.

13. How should frozen fruits be served? ___________________________
Fruits have the best flavor if served with a few ice crystals remaining.

14. How should frozen meat, poultry, and fish be thawed? Meat, poultry, and fish should be allowed to thaw overnight in a refrigerator or using the defrost setting on a microwave oven right before cooking.

15. How do you determine when partially thawed meat can be refrozen? If meat is partially thawed but still firm, it can be refrozen. If meat is fully thawed, it should not be refrozen.

Drying

Name _______________________________

Date _________________________ Period ___________

The steps for preparing, drying, and storing fruits and vegetables are listed below. Reorganize the lettered steps so they are in the correct order. Write the letters in the spaces that follow the numbers. Then answer the questions, writing your responses in the space provided.

Steps:

1. __I__   A. Allow vegetables to become hard and brittle and fruits to become leathery and pliable.

2. __L__   B. Blanch vegetables and sulfur fruits.

3. __D__   C. Make drying trays by tacking wire screening to a wooden frame.

4. __B__   D. Cut fruits and vegetables into small pieces.

5. __C__   E. Rotate trays and occasionally stir food to ensure even drying.

6. __J__   F. Package dried foods in insect-proof and moisture-proof containers.

7. __G__   G. Stack trays evenly in the oven, with the lower oven rack about 3 inches from the oven bottom.

8. __E__   H. Seal and label containers.

9. __A__   I. Select young, tender vegetables in prime condition and fruits at optimum maturity.

10. __F__   J. Spread food in a single layer on drying tray.

11. __H__   K. Store containers in a cool, dark place.

12. __K__   L. Wash fruits and vegetables.

13. Briefly explain how drying preserves food. Microorganisms that cause food spoilage need moisture to grow. Drying removes moisture, thus stopping the growth of microorganisms.

14. Why are dried foods popular with campers, cyclists, and backpackers? Dried foods are popular with campers, cyclists, and backpackers because they are lightweight and take up less space than fresh foods.

15. What treatment other than sulfuring can be used to keep fruit from darkening? A salt solution can be used to keep fruit from darkening.

16. Why should vegetables be cut into small pieces for drying? Smaller pieces dry more quickly and evenly.

17. What two appliances can be used to oven dry foods? Oven drying can be done in a food dehydrator or a conventional oven.

18. What is one advantage and one disadvantage of sun drying? Sun drying is less costly than oven drying, but it relies on the weather.

19. What types of containers are suitable for storing dried foods? Plastic containers, glass jars, and waxed cartons are all suitable for storing dried foods.

20. How are dried vegetables prepared for cooking? Rehydrate dried vegetables by soaking them in water for an hour or two. Simmer vegetables in the same water used for soaking until they are tender.

Shelf Life of Foods

<table>
<tr><td>Activity F</td><td>Name ___________________________</td></tr>
<tr><td>Chapter 25</td><td>Date _____________ Period _______</td></tr>
</table>

Give the shelf life for each of the following foods according to the type of storage indicated. Write your responses in the space provided.

Freezer Storage

1. Beef: 6 to 12 months
2. Bread: 2 to 3 months
3. Fish: 3 to 4 months
4. Frozen vegetables: 9 to 12 months
5. Ground meat: 3 months
6. Hot dogs: 2 months
7. Ice cream: 2 months
8. Lamb: 6 to 9 months
9. Pork: 3 to 6 months
10. Poultry: 6 to 8 months

Refrigerator Storage

11. Bacon: 5 to 7 days
12. Beef: 2 to 4 days
13. Natural cheese: 4 to 8 weeks
14. Fish: 1 to 2 days
15. Fresh fruit: varies according to type
16. Pork: 2 to 4 days
17. Poultry: 1 to 2 days
18. Fresh vegetables: varies according to type

Shelf Storage

19. Aseptically packaged juice: 6 months
20. Canned peaches: 1 year
21. Dried beans: 1 year
22. Flour: 1 year
23. Home-canned tomatoes: 1 year
24. Onions: 4 weeks
25. Raisins: 1 year

Investigating Careers

Pathway to Success

Activity A   **Name** ____

Chapter 26   **Date** ____________________________ **Period** _____________

Visit the O*Net Online website. Navigate the site to complete the following exercise about a career pathway of interest to you. Write your responses in the space provided.

1. Under *Find Occupations*, click on *Career Cluster*. From the drop-down menu, name the Career Cluster that most interests you and explain why. (Answers will vary.) _______________________

   ____

2. When you click on your chosen Career Cluster, a list of occupations appears sorted by career pathways. How many pathways are in your Career Cluster? (Answers will vary.) _______________

3. Review the pathways and associated occupations. Name the career pathway that most interests you and explain why.

   (Answers will vary.) ____

   ____

4. Name the occupation in your chosen career pathway that most interests you and explain why.

   (Answers will vary.) ____

   ____

5. Click on your chosen occupation. Complete the first and fourth columns in the following table with three types of knowledge and three skills needed for success in this occupation.

Knowledge	✓	✓	Skills	✓	✓
(Answers will vary.)					

6. Name a second occupation in your chosen career pathway that interests you. (Answers will vary.) ______

7. Click on your second chosen occupation. Place check marks in the second and fifth columns of the table above if listed types of knowledge and skills, respectively, are needed for success in this occupation.

8. Name a third occupation in your chosen career pathway that interests you. (Answers will vary.) ________

9. Click on your third chosen occupation. Place check marks in the third and sixth columns of the table above if listed types of knowledge and skills, respectively, are needed for success in this occupation.

10. What does this exercise reveal to you about knowledge and skills needed for success in occupations that interest you?

    (Answers will vary.) ____

    ____

Considering Career Options

Name _______________________________

Date _______________________ **Period** ___________

Answer the following questions to help you identify career options that match your interests.

1. What are two hobbies you enjoy? (Answers will vary.) ______________________

   ____

2. What are your two favorite subjects in school? (Answers will vary.) __________

   ____

3. How much would you expect to earn as a starting salary? (Answers will vary.)

   _____ less than $15,000   _____ $15,000 to $24,999   _____ $25,000 to $34,999

   _____ $35,000 to $49,999   _____ $50,000 or more

4. What is the highest educational recognition you plan to earn? (Answers will vary.)

   _____ high school diploma   _____ trade school/technical school certificate

   _____ associate's degree   _____ bachelor's degree   _____ master's degree   _____ doctoral degree

5. Do you expect to work full-time? (Answers will vary.) ______________________

   If not, explain why. (Answers will vary.) ________________________________

   ____

6. How frequently would you be willing to travel for work? (Answers will vary.)

   _____ not at all   _____ 2 to 3 times per year   _____ monthly   _____ 2 to 3 times per month

7. For each of the following pairs of personality traits, circle the one that best describes you.
   (Answers will vary.)

adventurous/cautious	honest/insincere	organized/messy
conservative/liberal	lighthearted/serious	outgoing/shy
frugal/extravagant	nervous/confident	particular/imprecise

8. Where would you prefer to live? (Answers will vary.) _____ _____ city _____ suburbs _____ country

9. What schedule would you be willing to work? (Check all that apply.) (Answers will vary.)

   _____ business hours (9 AM to 5 PM)   _____ first shift (6 AM to 2 PM)

   _____ second shift (2 PM to 10 PM)   _____ third shift (10 PM to 6 AM)

   _____ weekdays   _____ weekends

10. Review your answers to all the previous questions. Based on your review, what careers do you feel you are best suited to explore further? Explain your answer.

    (Answers will vary.)

    ____

    ____

    ____

Finding Career Information

Activity C   Name _______________________________________

Chapter 26   Date ______________________________ Period ____________

Answer the following questions to help identify resources you can use to learn more about careers. Write your responses in the space provided.

1. What are two questions you would like to ask your school counselor about careers and career preparation? (Answers will vary.) _______________________________

   ____

2. Which one of your teachers would be a good source of information about careers that interest you? Explain your answer. (Answers will vary.) ___________________________

   ____

3. How could your parents help you obtain career information? (Answers will vary.) ______

   ____

4. Who in your community is involved in careers that interest you? (Answers will vary.) ____

   What types of career information do you think you could obtain from these people?____

   (Answers will vary.) ____

5. Visit the websites of two postsecondary schools that offer curriculum related to your area of career interest.

   Which schools did you investigate? (Answers will vary.) ________________________

   What information did you learn about possible programs of study? (Answers will vary.) ___

   ____

   ____

6. What is a leading professional organization in your desired career field that would offer career information and announce job openings? (Answers will vary.) _________________

   ____

   What professional journal(s) does this organization publish? (Answers will vary.) _______

7. Visit three occupational information websites and explore the resources available at each site. List the sites you visited. (Answers will vary.) ___________________________

   ____

   Which site would you prefer to use to research careers? Explain your answer. (Answers will vary.) ____

   ____

   ____

8. Use a social networking site to search for information about three companies that interest you.

   What networking site did you use? (Answers will vary.) ________________________

   Which companies did you research? (Answers will vary.) _______________________

   ____

   What types of information were you able to learn? (Answers will vary.) ____________

   ____

You're the Boss

Name _______________________________

Date _______________________ **Period** ___________

Answer the following questions to help you explore your interest in becoming an entrepreneur. Write your responses in the space provided.

1. What types of products or services would your business provide? (Answers will vary.) ________

    ____

2. Where would your business be located? (Answers will vary.) _______________________

    ____

3. Why do you think this type of business would be successful in this location? (Answers will vary.) ____

    ____

4. Who would your customers be? (Answers will vary.) ___________________________

    ____

5. What other businesses would create competition for you? (Answers will vary.) ___________

    ____

6. What types of equipment and supplies would you need to purchase to operate this business? _______

    (Answers will vary.) ____

7. How many employees would you need to hire to help you run this business? What tasks would they perform? (Answers will vary.) ____

    ____

8. How much money do you think it would take to get this business started? (Do not forget to consider such expenses as rent, utilities, office supplies and equipment, accounting and legal fees, shipping and advertising costs, salaries, and taxes.) (Answers will vary.) ___________________

9. What kind of education would help you prepare to open this business? (Answers will vary.) _______

    ____

10. Where could you get work experience that would help you prepare to open this business? _________

    (Answers will vary.) ____

11. What would you name your business? (Answers will vary.) ________________________

12. How would you advertise your business? (Answers will vary.) _____________________

    ____

After answering the above questions, would you have any interest in further exploring entrepreneurship? Explain why or why not.

(Answers will vary.) ____

____

____

____

Career and Job Success

Performance Review

Activity A   Name ____

Chapter 27   Date ____________________________ Period ____________

Imagine you are the operations manager of a moderate-sized company. At their annual performance reviews, you want to provide the following employees with constructive criticism. In the space provided, write what you would say to each employee to affirm his or her strengths. Then explain why and how he or she might make changes to improve his or her job performance.

1. Wendy is responsible for opening and delivering the mail to everyone in the office. She stops to have a friendly chat with each person to whom she delivers mail. You have noticed it has been taking Wendy longer and longer to complete this task each day.

   (Answers will vary.)

   ____

   ____

2. You see Tim working late one evening. He is busily making numerous photocopies, folding and stuffing the copies into envelopes, and running the envelopes through the mail meter. When you ask Tim what he is working on, he tells you he is copying and sending 100 letters to request support for his daughter's charity event.

   (Answers will vary.)

   ____

   ____

3. Dana is not part of the custodial staff. However, she spends about 15 minutes after lunch each day cleaning up in the break room before returning to her desk.

   (Answers will vary.)

   ____

   ____

4. Kenneth always seems to know about the latest research. He reads every article in every professional journal that lands in his inbox. However, he is frequently late turning in mandatory reports and time sheets.

   (Answers will vary.)

   ____

   ____

(Continued)

5. Jalisa works at the reception desk greeting clients when they enter your building. She never engages in small talk as she efficiently gathers information from clients and answers any questions they might have. More than once, clients have commented that Jalisa is *all business*.

(Answers will vary.)

6. Donny works in your warehouse loading and unloading trucks. Although he does not interact directly with clients, he does bring packages into the front office from time to time. Donny is a good worker, but he always looks like he just rolled out of bed. He never seems to comb his hair, and his jeans and T-shirts always look stained and dingy.

(Answers will vary.)

7. Clarence is another warehouse worker. He is your fastest worker when it comes to packing and shipping orders. In his haste, however, he often drives the forklift too fast and forgets to wear his hardhat.

(Answers will vary.)

8. Cindy's job is to type survey responses into data fields on a computer. Her work is always complete and error free. However, she asks her supervisor for help every time she runs into a nonstandard response on one of the surveys.

(Answers will vary.)

9. Carl takes more phone orders from customers than any of your other salespeople. However, he also has the highest percentage of order returns. You have observed that Carl's high-volume sales technique involves quickly talking customers into your most popular product whenever they seem uncertain about what to order.

(Answers will vary.)

10. Terrence is never shy about taking charge at team brainstorming meetings. In fact, he offers so many ideas that some of the other team members feel there is no need for them to make suggestions.

(Answers will vary.)

Letter of Resignation

Activity B   Name _______________________________________

Chapter 27   Date _____________________________ Period ______________

Your friend tells you she plans to walk off her job tomorrow because she is sick of the work and fed up with her boss. You talk her into writing a letter of resignation, so she gives you the following letter to review. In the space following the letter, write the suggestions you would give your friend for rewriting her letter.

> Dear Mason,
>
> I wanted you to know that I am quiting at the end of the week. I can't stand working for you anymore. You don't pay enough attention to notice how hard I work and pay me what I'm worth.
>
> Sincerly,
>
> Komali

(Answers will vary.)

Balancing Multiple Roles

Activity C   Name ___________________________

Chapter 27   Date _____________________   Period ____________

Read each of the scenarios that follow and answer the questions in the space provided.

1. John is scheduled to help train a new employee tomorrow afternoon. He just received a call from his daughter saying she is receiving an award at school tomorrow at 2:30 p.m.

   What roles does John need to balance in this situation? *employee, parent*

   What would you do if you were John? *(Answers will vary.)*

2. Jamie just got home from the office with a briefcase full of reports she needs to review for a meeting tomorrow. She finds that her husband isn't feeling well and needs her to go pick up a prescription for him. Then Jamie sees there are two loads of laundry waiting to be folded, and someone needs to get dinner started.

   What roles does Jamie need to balance in this situation? *employee, spouse, homemaker*

   What would you do if you were Jamie? *(Answers will vary.)*

3. Maritza had agreed to call local businesses this week to ask for donations for a charity fund-raiser. Then her employer asked her to work double shifts all week to cover for a vacationing coworker. Maritza also promised to visit her grandmother at the nursing home this week.

   What roles does Maritza need to balance in this situation? *citizen, employee, granddaughter*

   What would you do if you were Maritza? *(Answers will vary.)*

4. Trevor has been offered a promotion, but taking it would mean moving his family to another city. Trevor's wife is a manager at a local department store. His children are in second and third grade. Trevor and his wife are very involved in their church, and Trevor coaches his son's soccer team.

   What roles does Trevor need to balance in this situation? *employee, spouse, parent, citizen*

   What would you do if you were Trevor? *(Answers will vary.)*

5. Malcolm is scheduled to work at *Bonanza Burger* this evening. Before he goes into work, Malcolm needs to clean his room and study for a test. He also promised his sister he would help her with her math homework. Then a few friends called and asked him to come out and shoot some hoops.

   What roles does Malcolm need to balance in this situation? *employee, son, student, brother, friend*

   What would you do if you were Malcolm? *(Answers will vary.)*

The United States and Canada

A Holiday Celebration

Activity A   **Name** _______________________________________

Chapter 28   **Date** _____________________________ **Period** ___________

Presume you own the *Green Roof Inn*. The inn is always busy, but it is especially popular with families during holidays. Answer the following questions about how you will create a unique holiday celebration package for your guests. Write your responses in the space provided.

1. For which holiday are you planning? (Answers will vary.) ___________________________

2. What event does this holiday celebrate? (Answers will vary.) _______________________

   ____

3. What is the name of the holiday package? (Answers will vary.) _____________________

4. When will this package be offered? (Answers will vary.) ___________________________

5. Other than overnight accommodations and a special meal, what will the package include?

   (Answers will vary.) ____

   ____

6. What regional or cultural traditions are part of this holiday celebration in your area? How can you include some of these traditions in the celebration at the Green Roof Inn?

   (Answers will vary.) ____

   ____

7. What activities will you plan to entertain the children of your guests? ________________

   (Answers will vary.) ____

   ____

8. Write a menu of the foods you will serve your guests for the special holiday meal that is part of their package. (Answers will vary.) _______________________________________

   ____

   ____

   ____

9. Why did you choose the foods you did? (Answers will vary.) _______________________

   ____

10. What do you hope will be the most memorable part of your guests' holiday celebration at the Green Roof Inn? (Answers will vary.) ______________________________________

   ____

Cultural Influences on Food

Activity B   Name ____

Chapter 28   Date ______________________________   Period ____________

Select a region from the following map and use markers or colored pencils to color it. Then answer the questions regarding food customs in that region in the space provided. If necessary, use an additional sheet of paper for your answers and attach it to this activity.

Region: (Answers will vary.) ____

1. What group(s) of people settled this region? (Answers will vary.) ____________

   ____

2. What foods are native to this region? (Answers will vary.) ________________

   ____

3. How did the settlers use these native foods to prepare the dishes of their homeland(s)?__________

   (Answers will vary.) ____

4. What foods were introduced by the settlers? (Answers will vary.) ___________

   ____

5. What cooking methods were used by the settlers? (Answers will vary.) ________

   ____

6. How did cultural customs and traditions affect the types of foods and cooking methods used by the settlers? (Answers will vary.) ____________________________________

   ____

7. What dishes introduced by the settlers are still typical of this region today? (Answers will vary.) ____

   ____

8. How do dishes typically served in this region today reflect the culture of the people who settled the region? (Answers will vary.) ____________________________________

   ____

Regional Foods Match

Activity C   Name ______________________________________

Chapter 28   Date ___________________________   Period _____________

Match the regions of the United States with the letters of the foods typical of each region. (There are three matches for each region.) Write the letters of the correct responses in the space provided.

A. sopapillas
B. andouille
C. sourdough bread
D. barbecued beef short ribs
E. caribou sausage
F. kalua puaa
G. shoofly pie

H. corn on the cob
I. succotash
J. poi
K. macadamia nuts
L. baked beans
M. jambalaya
N. scrapple

O. chitterlings
P. apple pie
Q. broiled steak
R. clam chowder
S. salmon steaks
T. chicken corn soup
U. tamales

_I_   _L_   _R_   1. New England
_G_   _N_   _T_   2. Mid-Atlantic
_B_   _M_   _O_   3. South
_H_   _P_   _Q_   4. Midwest
_A_   _D_   _U_   5. West and Southwest
_C_   _E_   _S_   6. Pacific Coast
_F_   _J_   _K_   7. Hawaiian Islands

8. List the groups of people who influenced the cuisines in each region of the United States.

   A. New England: British

   B. Mid-Atlantic: Dutch, Germans, Swedes, British

   C. South: French, British, Irish, Scots, Spaniards, African slaves, Native Americans

   D. Midwest: Swedes, Greeks, Germans, Poles, Italians

   E. West and Southwest: Native Americans, Mexicans, Spaniards, cowboys

   F. Pacific Coast: Chinese, Japanese, Koreans, Polynesians, Mexicans, prospectors

   G. Hawaiian Islands: Polynesians, Europeans, Chinese, Japanese

        Chapter 28   The United States and Canada

Create a Canadian Menu

Activity D   **Name** ___________________________________

Chapter 28   **Date** _________________________ **Period** ___________

Answer the following questions as you plan a menu that reflects the ingredients and food customs of Canada. Remember to keep variety of flavors, colors, textures, shapes, sizes, and temperatures in mind as you select foods for your menu. Write your responses in the space provided.

1. For what meal will this menu be served? (Answers will vary.)

2. What are you serving for your first course/appetizer? (Answers will vary.)

   What are the main ingredients in this dish? (Answers will vary.)

   Why is this dish a good example of Canadian cuisine? (Answers will vary.)

3. What are you serving for your main dish? (Answers will vary.)

   What are the main ingredients in this dish? (Answers will vary.)

   Why is this dish a good example of Canadian cuisine? (Answers will vary.)

4. What are you serving for a starchy side dish? (Answers will vary.)

   What are the main ingredients in this dish? (Answers will vary.)

   Why is this dish a good example of Canadian cuisine? (Answers will vary.)

5. What are you serving for a vegetable? (Answers will vary.)

   What are the main ingredients in this dish? (Answers will vary.)

   Why is this dish a good example of Canadian cuisine? (Answers will vary.)

6. What are you serving for a salad? (Answers will vary.)

   What are the main ingredients in this dish? (Answers will vary.)

   Why is this dish a good example of Canadian cuisine? (Answers will vary.)

7. What are you serving for dessert? (Answers will vary.)

   What are the main ingredients in this dish? (Answers will vary.)

   Why is this dish a good example of Canadian cuisine? (Answers will vary.)

8. What are you serving to drink? (Answers will vary.)

   Why is this beverage a good example of Canadian cuisine? (Answers will vary.)

9. What else, if anything, are you serving with this meal? (Answers will vary.)

   How do these foods reflect Canadian cuisine? (Answers will vary.)

Latin America

Mexican Cuisine

Activity A   Name ____

Chapter 29   Date _______________________   Period ____________

The foods in the following list are all important in Mexican cuisine. For each item, if the food was contributed by the Aztecs, write *A* in the blank to the left of the number. If the food was contributed by the Spanish, write *S* in the blank. Then answer the questions that follow.

_A_	1. peppers		_S_	9. rice
_S_	2. chicken		_A_	10. beans
_S_	3. wheat		_A_	11. tomatoes
_A_	4. chocolate		_S_	12. beef
_S_	5. peaches		_S_	13. cinnamon
_A_	6. corn		_S_	14. oil
_A_	7. vanilla		_A_	15. squash
_A_	8. pineapples		_A_	16. avocados

17. Name three staple ingredients in Mexican cuisine. Describe a dish made with each of the ingredients.

    Corn. (Answers will vary.)

    Beans. (Answers will vary.)

    Peppers. (Answers will vary.)

18. List three vegetables and three fruits grown in Mexico. Describe one Mexican fruit or vegetable dish.

    Vegetables: (List three:) zucchini, artichokes, white potatoes, spinach, chard, lettuce, beets, cauliflower, carrots, huazontle, jicama, nopole, chayotes

    Fruits: (List three:) avocados, bananas, pineapples, guavas, papayas, prickly pears

    Fruit or vegetable dish: (Answers will vary.)

19. Identify two regions of Mexico and describe a dish typical of each region.

    A. (Answers will vary.)

    B. (Answers will vary.)

20. Name two meals served in Mexico and describe foods typically served at those meals.

    A. (Answers will vary.)

    B. (Answers will vary.)

Mexico Q and A

<table>
<tr><td>Activity B</td><td>Name ___________________________________</td></tr>
<tr><td>Chapter 29</td><td>Date _____________________   Period __________</td></tr>
</table>

Imagine you have just returned from a trip to Mexico. The editor of your company newsletter wants to write an article about your trip for the next edition. In the space provided, write your responses to the following interview questions asked by the editor.

Q: Mexico is part of the landmass known as Latin America. Can you tell me why it is called this?

A: 1. The landmass that stretches southward from the Rio Grande to the tip of South America is called Latin America because the official language of most of the countries is either Spanish or Portuguese, both of which are based on Latin.

Q: Many people travel to Mexico to get a break from cold winter weather. What is the climate like in Mexico?

A: 2. Although the climate in a few regions is wet and humid, nearly half of Mexico is arid or semiarid.

Q: I'm sure the Mexican landscape offers far more than the beaches shown in many travel brochures. How would you describe the geography of Mexico?

A: 3. Much of Mexico is mountainous with valleys separating the different ranges.

Q: I understand climate and geography have both had an influence on the cuisine of Mexico. Can you give me one example?

A: 4. (Answers will vary.)

Q: I would like our readers to form a clear mental picture of the lifestyle of Mexico. What do furnishings in a typical Mexican home look like?

A: 5. Beds, tables, and chairs often are hand-carved. Many dishes and cooking utensils are handmade.

(Continued)

Q: The majority of people in the United States work in service industries. Could you describe what kind of work most Mexican people do?

A: 6. A little more than half of Mexico's people are farmers.

Q: Chief agricultural products of the United States include beef, cattle, cotton, soybeans, and wheat. What key agricultural products come from Mexico?

A: 7. Corn is Mexico's major crop. Bean production is second. Other important crops include sugarcane, coffee, tomatoes, green peppers, peas, melons, citrus fruits, strawberries, and cacao beans.

Q: Many people in the United States are concerned about the nutritional value of their food. How would you describe the nutritional quality of Mexican foods?

A: 8. (Answers will vary.)

Q: Most people in the United States are familiar with tacos and enchiladas as foods that are common throughout Mexico. What types of dishes are more characteristic of the coastal region you visited?

A: 9. (Answers will vary.)

Q: We generally eat breakfast, lunch, and dinner with a few between-meal snacks. How do Mexican meals differ from this?

A: 10. Mexican families with ample incomes eat four meals a day. *Desayuno* is a substantial breakfast. *Comida*, the main meal of the day, is served between one and three o'clock. *Merienda* is a light snack served around five or six o'clock. *Cena*, or supper, is eaten between eight and 10 o'clock.

South American Culture and Cuisine

Activity C Name _______________________________

Chapter 29 Date _____________________ Period ___________

Identify each of the South American countries indicated on the map. Match each food listed below with the country to which it is most associated. Then provide a brief description of how the food is served or used.

ajiaco   dendé oil
arepa   papa
bananas   pastel de choclo
chimichurri

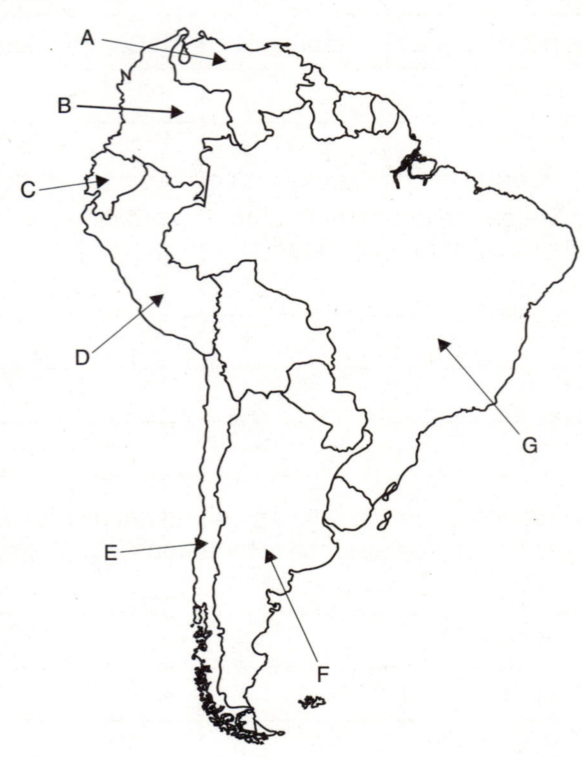

A. Country: Venezuela

   Food: arepa

   (Answers will vary.)

B. Country: Colombia

   Food: ajiaco

   (Answers will vary.)

C. Country: Ecuador

   Food: bananas

   (Answers will vary.)

D. Country: Peru

   Food: papa

   (Answers will vary.)

E. Country: Chile

   Food: pastel de choclo

   (Answers will vary.)

F. Country: Argentina

   Food: chimichurri

   (Answers will vary.)

G. Country: Brazil

   Food: dendé oil

   (Answers will vary.)

CHAPTER 30
Europe

British Culture and Cuisine

Activity A   Name ____

Chapter 30   Date _______________________________ Period _____________

1. Label the five countries indicated on the map of the British Isles.

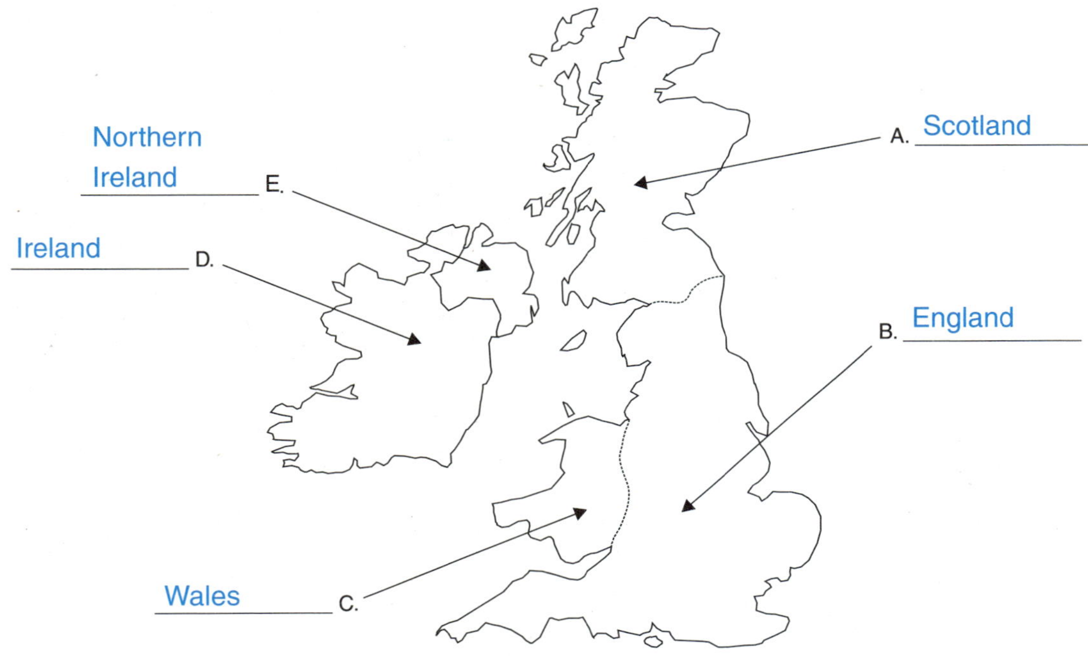

Match the countries in the map with each of the following words or phrases about British culture and cuisine. Place the letter of the country that is most closely associated with each word or phrase in the blank provided to the left of the number.

__A__	2. wassail bowl		__A__	15. Highland games
__C__	3. cawl		__A__	16. Hogmanay
__C__	4. Brecon Beacons		__B__	17. land o the Angles
__A__	5. cock-a-leekie		__E__	18. part of the United Kingdom not on the island of Great Britain
__C__	6. cockles			
__D, E__	7. corned beef and cabbage		__D, E__	19. potatoes
__C__	8. crempog		__B__	20. shepherd's pie
__D__	9. Eire		__D, E__	21. soda bread
__A__	10. finnan haddie		__C__	22. St. David's Day
__B__	11. fish and chips		__B__	23. steamed puddings
__D__	12. Gaelic is an official language		__E__	24. strife between Protestants and Catholics
__B__	13. Guy Fawkes Night			
__A__	14. haggis		__C__	25. tatws sla

France Crossword

Name _______________________________________

Date _______________________________ Period _____________

Across

2. At breakfast, the French often drink hot milk and coffee, or _______ au lait.
4. A rare type of fungi that grow underground near oak trees are called _______.
8. Small dishes designed to stimulate the appetite are called _______.
9. The French cuisine enjoyed by most French families, which features locally grown foods and simple cooking methods, is _______.
11. A custard tart that originated in the Lorraine region is known as _______.
13. Brittany is known for thin, delicate, filled pancakes called _______.
14. A specialty of the Burgundy region is snails eaten as food, which are known as _______.
16. A famous dish in Burgundy that is flavored with local wine is _______ á la Bourguignonne.

Down

1. Flaky, buttery yeast rolls shaped into crescents are called _______.
3. Many dishes of the Rhône-_______ region combine three staple foods—potatoes, milk, and cheese.
5. A mixture of fresh chives, parsley, tarragon, and chervil is called _______.
6. A French cuisine that emphasizes lightness and natural taste in foods is _______.
7. The second Sunday in May is a French holiday that honors Joan of _______.
9. Finely chopped and seasoned meat of game birds, such as pigeons, is made into a spread called _______.
10. The French call Christmas _______.
12. A French cuisine characterized by elaborate preparations, fancy garnishes, and rich sauces is _______.
15. A mixture of butter (or other fat) and flour that forms the base of white sauces used in French cooking is called a _______.

Foods of Germany

Activity C Name _______________________________

Chapter 30 Date _______________________ Period ___________

Choose from among the following words to fill in the blanks and complete the statements below about German foods.

braten	hasenpfeffer	pumpernickel	schnitzel
bratwurst	kartoffelpuffer	salzkartoffeln	spätzle
braunschweiger	kasseler rippenspeer	sauerbraten	stollen
eintopf	lebkuchen	sauerkraut	strudel
gebildbrote	preiselbeeren	schinkenwurst	Westphalian ham

1. _Bratwurst_ is a sausage made of freshly ground, seasoned pork that is usually cooked by grilling.

2. Small dumplings made from wheat flour called _spätzle_ are a popular German side dish.

3. _Hasenpfeffer_ is a rabbit dish that is braised in a marinade of wine, vinegar, onions, and spices.

4. Small, cranberry-like fruits called _preiselbeeren_ are often served with game dishes.

5. _Westphalian ham_ is a richly flavored, smoked uncooked ham that is served throughout Germany.

6. Young men and women sometimes give the honey-spice cake called _lebkuchen_ to their sweethearts as gifts.

7. _Kasseler rippenspeer_ is a whole smoked pork loin that is roasted and served with sauerkraut, apples or chestnuts, peas, white beans, mushrooms, and browned potatoes.

8. _Sauerkraut_ is fermented or pickled cabbage that is usually flavored with caraway, apple, onion, or juniper berries and served with pork dishes.

9. _Braunschweiger_ is a type of liver sausage that was first produced in Braunschweig, Germany.

10. _Schnitzel_ is a breaded, sautéed veal cutlet.

11. At Christmastime, Germans may serve a rich yeast bread called _stollen_, which is filled with almonds, raisins, and candied fruit.

12. _Pumpernickel_ bread, made from unsifted rye flour, is a favorite in Germany.

13. _Sauerbraten_, a sweet-sour marinated beef roast, is a popular beef dish in Germany.

14. A German dessert made with paper-thin layers of pastry filled with plums, apples, cherries, or poppy seeds is called _strudel_.

15. _Kartoffelpuffer_ are the famous potato pancakes enjoyed throughout Germany.

16. Breads baked into fanciful shapes are called _gebildbrote_, which means picture breads.

17. _Salzkartoffeln_ are potatoes cooked in salted water that are drained and steamed until dry.

18. Leftover meats are used to make _eintopf_, a popular stew.

Influences on Scandinavian Cuisine

Activity D   **Name** ______________________________

Chapter 30   **Date** ____________________   **Period** __________

Use complete sentences to answer the following questions about Scandinavian climate, geography, and cuisine. Write your responses in the space provided.

1. A. Briefly describe the seasonal climate of Norway, Sweden, and Finland. ______________
   Winters in Norway, Sweden, and Finland are long and severe. Summers are short and cool.

   B. How has climate affected food production in these countries? ______________________
   The growing season in Norway, Sweden, and Finland is short so agricultural production is limited.

   C. How has climate affected food preservation in these countries? Careful preservation of food is
   important in Norway, Sweden, and Finland. Pickled, dried, and salted foods are common.

2. A. Briefly describe the geography of Norway, Sweden, and Finland. The geography of Norway,
   Sweden, and Finland is rugged. Norway has a mountainous coast. Much of northern Sweden is
   covered by forests. Finland is stony with many lakes and marshy areas.

   B. How has geography affected food production in these countries? ____________________
   Only a small percentage of the land in Norway, Sweden, and Finland can be farmed.

3. How does Denmark's climate differ from that of the other Scandinavian countries? ________
   Denmark is mild with plenty of rainfall. The winters are warmer than in other Scandinavian countries.

4. How does Denmark's geography differ from that of the other Scandinavian countries? Denmark's land
   is less rugged. Forests fringe the eastern shore and hills cut through the central part of the country.

5. How do climate and geography affect food production in Denmark? ____________________
   Denmark has a longer growing season than the other Scandinavian countries and about 75 percent
   of the land can be farmed.

6. What industry is important to all four Scandinavian countries? ______________________
   Fishing is an important industry to all four Scandinavian countries.

7. What are Denmark's main agricultural products? ________________________________
   Denmark's main agricultural products come from pigs, cows, and chickens.

8. What are the main agricultural products of the other Scandinavian countries? Grain and livestock are
   the main agricultural products of Norway, Sweden, and Finland. Norway also produces potatoes.

9. How does Danish cuisine differ from that of the other Scandinavian countries? Danish food is richer
   than that of the other Scandinavian countries due to the use of large quantities of butter, cream, cheese,
   and eggs. Fish is not as popular in Denmark as in the other countries. Danes eat more pork and chicken.

10. Give an example with a brief description of a dish typical of each of the Scandinavian countries.
    A. Denmark: (Answers will vary.)
    B. Norway: (Answers will vary.)
    C. Sweden: (Answers will vary.)
    D. Finland: (Answers will vary.)

Cuisine Travel Guide

Activity E　　　　　　**Name** ______________________________________

Chapter 30　　　　　　**Date** _______________________　　**Period** ______________

Imagine you are a travel agent. Part of your job involves designing travel brochures for a *Cuisines of Europe* travel package your company is offering. On these pages, design a travel brochure for one of the European countries. Use information from the text and other resources to provide some background on the country. Then focus on the cuisine so people will want to visit the country. Place drawings or pictures from newspapers, magazines, or the Internet in the boxes to illustrate your brochure. Use your creativity to develop a descriptive, interesting brochure rather than just a fact sheet.

Country: (Answers will vary.) ______________________________________

Climate (Answers will vary.) __________________________________

____

____

Geography (Answers will vary.) _______________________________

____

____

Size: (Answers will vary.) _______________________________

Capital city: (Answers will vary.) ________________________

General Information

Population: (Answers will vary.) __________________________

Language spoken: (Answers will vary.) ____________________

Historical background: (Answers will vary.) ________________

____

____

____

Form of government: (Answers will vary.) __________________

Primary religion: (Answers will vary.) _____________________

Major industries: (Answers will vary.) _____________________

____

(Continued)

Customs and beliefs: (Answers will vary.)

Native costume: (Answers will vary.)

Holidays: (Answers will vary.)

Points of interest: (Answers will vary.)

Cuisine

Common ingredients: (Answers will vary.)

Typical dishes (list five, describe two): (Answers will vary.)

Characteristics of the cuisine: (Answers will vary.)

Preparation methods: (Answers will vary.)

Meal patterns: (Answers will vary.)

Serving customs: (Answers will vary.)

Mediterranean Countries

Spanish Culture and Cuisine

Activity A Name _______________________________

Chapter 31 Date _______________________ Period ____________

Match the following descriptions related to the culture and cuisine of Spain with the terms they describe. Place the correct letter in the corresponding blank to the left of each number.

___L___	1. This large plateau occupies more than half of Spain.	A. all-i-oli
___I___	2. Many Spaniards make their living in these industries.	B. almuerzo
___Y___	3. These Spanish-grown fruits are among the best in the world.	C. banderillas
___D___	4. This is part of the festivities during the annual feast day observed for the patron saint of each town.	D. bullfight
___H___	5. This term, which means food of the people, describes Spanish cuisine.	E. buñelitos
___O___	6. The Romans contributed these ingredients to Spanish cuisine.	F. chorizo
___N___	7. These people crossed into Spain from Africa in A.D. 711, bringing many cultural and culinary advances.	G. cocido
___M___	8. Spanish cooking should not be confused with the spicy cooking of this country.	H. del pueblo
___S___	9. This Spanish sauce is flavored and colored with large amounts of parsley.	I. fishing and farming
___G___	10. Vegetables, beef, lamb, ham, poultry, and a spicy sausage cook together in a large pot to make this dish.	J. flan
___W___	11. These are Spanish appetizers.	K. gazpacho
___E___	12. These small pieces of vegetables, meat, poultry, or fish are battered, deep-fried, and served as appetizers.	L. Meseta
___Q___	13. These grilled foods are served as appetizers.	M. Mexico
___V___	14. This is a fish soup in which all the ingredients are cooked together for 15 minutes.	N. Moors
___K___	15. This soup is often made with coarsely pureed tomatoes, onions, garlic, and green peppers; olive oil; and vinegar.	O. olive oil and garlic
___A___	16. This garlic mayonnaise is served with seafood in some parts of Spain.	P. paella
___F___	17. This dark sausage has a spicy, smoky flavor.	Q. pinchos
___P___	18. This Spanish rice dish has many variations.	R. pulses
___X___	19. This is a Spanish omelet.	S. salsa verde
___R___	20. The Spanish use this term to refer to dried beans, lentils, and chickpeas.	T. sangria
___J___	21. This caramel custard is a popular Spanish dessert.	U. sherry
___B___	22. This second morning meal is served at around 11 o'clock.	V. sopa al cuarto de hora
___U___	23. This popular Spanish wine has a nutlike flavor.	W. tapas
___T___	24. This wine-based punch is served throughout Spain.	X. tortilla
		Y. Valencian oranges

Italian Foods Identification

Identify each of the following Italian foods. Write *S* in the blank to the left of the number if the food is a type of seafood. Write *H* in the blank if the food is an herb. Write *P* in the blank if the food is a type of pasta. Write *C* in the blank if the food is a cheese. Then answer the questions that follow.

_C_	1. Parmesan		_H_	13. marjoram
_P_	2. orecchietta		_P_	14. cannelloni
_P_	3. fusilli		_C_	15. Romano
_H_	4. tarragon		_C_	16. ricotta
_C_	5. mozzarella		_P_	17. spaghetti
_S_	6. sardines		_S_	18. anchovies
_H_	7. oregano		_C_	19. provolone
_S_	8. sole		_H_	20. parsley
_P_	9. ricci di donna		_H_	21. thyme
_H_	10. sage		_C_	22. Gorgonzola
_S_	11. mussels		_S_	23. squid
_S_	12. oysters		_P_	24. lasagna

25. A. How do the pastas served in Northern Italy differ from those served in Southern Italy? __________
    In Northern Italy, pasta bolognese are served. These fat, ribbon-shaped pastas are usually made at home and contain egg. In Southern Italy, pasta napoletania are served. These tubular-shaped pastas are usually produced commercially and do not contain egg.

    B. Describe a dish that is a specialty of Northern Italy. (Answers will vary.)

    C. Describe a dish that is a specialty of Central Italy. (Answers will vary.)

    D. Describe a dish that is a specialty of Southern Italy. (Answers will vary.)

Italian Culture and Cuisine

Activity C   Name _______________________________

Chapter 31   Date _____________________________   Period __________

Read the following statements about Italian culture and cuisine. Circle *T* if the statement is true. Circle *F* if the statement is false.

(T) F   1. The most productive farming area in Italy is the Po River Valley, which is located in the northern part of the country.

T **(F)**   2. Southern Italy is the richest part of the country in terms of natural resources.

(T) F   3. Almost all Italians are Roman Catholics.

T **(F)**   4. Italians serve veal for Pasqua as a symbol of spring.

(T) F   5. Some Italian villages hold olive and fishing festivals in the late summer and early fall.

(T) F   6. During the Renaissance period, Italian cooking became the "mother cuisine"—the source of many other western cuisines

(T) F   7. The Greeks colonized Sicily and Southern Italy.

(T) F   8. Italy laid the foundation for French haute cuisine.

T **(F)**   9. Italian cooks rely heavily on convenience foods.

T **(F)**   10. Italian foods are bland because herbs and spices are seldom used.

T **(F)**   11. Many Italian foods are baked or roasted in the oven.

(T) F   12. Pasta, a paste made from wheat flour that is dried in various shapes, is eaten throughout Italy.

(T) F   13. Pasta should be served al dente, or slightly resistant to the bite.

(T) F   14. Because of the vast coastline of Italy, seafood is one of the Italian staple foods.

(T) F   15. The Italians introduced ice cream to the rest of Europe.

(T) F   16. Wine often replaces water at Italian meals.

T **(F)**   17. Northern Italian foods are spicy.

(T) F   18. Southern Italian cooking is the cooking with which most people in the United States are familiar.

(T) F   19. In Northern Italy, rice dishes called risottos may replace pasta at meals.

(T) F   20. A Northern Italian specialty is pollo alla cacciatore.

T **(F)**   21. Foods with Roman origins are specialties of Northern Italy.

T **(F)**   22. Spaghetti is seldom served in Rome.

(T) F   23. Cheesecake was invented by the Romans.

(T) F   24. Southern Italian dishes feature rich tomato sauces.

T **(F)**   25. Antipasto is the dessert course of an Italian meal.

The Greek Emporium

Activity D Name ______________________________

Chapter 31 Date ____________________ Period ____________

Pretend you work at The Greek Emporium, which is a specialty shop that sells foods and items imported from Greece. Patrons of the shop frequently ask questions not only about your merchandise, but about Greece in general. The owner hired you because your knowledge of Greece would help you answer these questions. Indicate how you would respond to each of the customer inquiries described below.

1. Mrs. Gremelli is planning a trip to Greece next winter. She is not sure what types of clothes she will need to buy for her trip. She wants to know what the terrain in Greece is like. She also wants to know what the weather in Greece is like during the winter months.

   Much of the land is a contrast of mountains and fertile valleys. Greece has mild, frost-free winters

   with some rainfall.

   ____

   ____

2. Mr. Addison enjoys eating at different ethnic restaurants. He recently made his first visit to a Greek restaurant. He was surprised to see olives offered as an appetizer on the menu. He also had not expected so many of the entrées to feature lamb and seafood. He wants to know why olives, lamb, and seafood seem to be so important in Greek cuisine.

   Greece is surrounded by water on three sides, making seafood widely available. The stony, dry soil

   in Greece is suitable for the cultivation of olive trees. Therefore, olives are a staple of Greek cuisine.

   Sheep thrive on the short grasses of the mountainous areas of Greece, causing lamb to be a

   common meat on Greek tables.

3. Mr. Pendant sees a display of Greek greeting cards in the shop. He notices many of the cards have religious symbols on them. He wants to know about the religion and holiday celebrations of the Greek people.

   The majority of Greeks belong to the Greek Orthodox Church. Religious holidays hold great

   importance for the Greek people. Easter is the most important religious holiday. The Greek people

   also celebrate Saint Basil's Day, which falls on New Year's Day, and a yearly feast day for the patron

   saint of their particular village or town. Some communities also hold annual harvest festivals.

4. Ms. Campbell picks up a musical instrument that looks like a mandolin. She wants to know what it is called and how it is used in Greek culture.

   The mandolin-like instrument is called a bouzoukia. In the evenings when people gather in the Greek

   tavernas, someone may play a bouzoukia while other guests talk, play games, or dance.

   ____

   ____

5. Mrs. Vander Meer is looking through the rack of books on Ancient Greece. She notices that most of the books have sizable sections on city-states. She wants to know what city-states were and what became of them.

   City-states were self-governing political units consisting of a city and surrounding territory. They

   eventually fell to the Roman Empire.

   ____

   ____

(Continued)

6. Mrs. Liang is browsing through your section of Greek cookbooks. She finds one titled *Hesiod's Fare*. She wants to know what this curious title means. She also wants to know what herbs and spices are commonly used in Greek cuisine.

   Hesiod was a Greek who wrote one of the first cookbooks. The most widely used herbs and spices in Greek cuisine include cinnamon, basil, dill, bay leaves, garlic, and oregano.

7. Mrs. Hiller loves to sample foods she has never tried before. She brings a packet of avgolemono sauce mix to the register. She wants to know what ingredients are in the sauce. She also wants to know how the sauce is used in Greek cuisine.

   Avgolemono is a mixture of egg yolks and lemon juice. The Greeks use it to flavor soups and stews. They also serve it with vegetables and fish.

8. Mr. Sanchez notices the emporium carries several varieties of Greek honey. He wants to know if Greek chefs really use much honey in their cooking. He wonders if you can tell him some specific Greek dishes that are prepared with honey.

   Honey is the basic sweetener used in the preparation of many Greek desserts. Greek bakers use it to make honey cakes to celebrate the New Year. They also use it in baklava and galatoboureko, two desserts made with the paper-thin pastry called *phyllo*.

9. Ms. Hodge sees packages of phyllo in the small freezer case in the back of the store. She says she knows phyllo is used to make baklava. She wants to know about some other dishes made with phyllo.

   Phyllo is used to make galatoboureko, which is phyllo layered with rich custard and honey. It is also used to make kopenhai, which is a nut cake with phyllo.

10. Mr. Masters notices it is nearly six o'clock and the shop will be closing soon. He says he is heading home to eat dinner. He wants to know if people in Greece eat dinner at this time of evening and what foods they typically serve.

    No, dinner in Greece is served late in the evening and might include baked or broiled fish, a vegetable, bread, and fresh fruit. In the early evening, people are more likely to gather at outdoor cafes. Here they enjoy a variety of appetizers called mezedhes along with ouzo and conversation.

Mediterranean Climate, Geography, and Cuisine

Activity E   **Name** ____

Chapter 31   **Date** _________________________   **Period** ____________

Complete the following chart by briefly describing the climate, geography, and cuisine of the Mediterranean countries discussed in the text. Then answer the questions that follow the chart.

Country	Climate	Geography	Cuisine
Spain			
Italy			
Greece			

What similarities exist among the three countries?

Climate: _(Answers will vary.)_______________________________________

Geography: _(Answers will vary.)_____________________________________

Cuisine: _(Answers will vary.)____

Middle East and Africa

Middle East Match

Activity A   Name ____

Chapter 32   Date _________________________________   Period ____________

Match the following descriptions related to the culture and cuisine of the Middle East with the terms they describe by writing the correct letters in the blanks to the left of the corresponding number.

A. bread	H. garlic	O. olive oil
B. bulgur	I. goats	P. Persian
C. coffee	J. green pepper	Q. Ramadan
D. cucumber	K. Halal	R. sheep
E. dolmas	L. irrigation	S. spices and herbs
F. eggplant	M. Islam	T. tea
G. Euphrates	N. lemon	U. tomato

G   1. Rich farm land is found along the banks of this Middle Eastern river.

L   2. This is an essential means of watering the dry lands of the Middle East.

P   3. This was the first of the four greatest empires that once flourished in the Middle East.

R   4. Middle Eastern herders raise these animals as the staple source of meat as well as for milk and hides.

M   5. This is the religion practiced by 90 percent of the people living in the Middle East.

Q   6. This is the ninth month of the Muslim calendar, during which a fast is observed throughout each day.

F,H,J,N,U   7. These five fruits and vegetables are basic to all Middle Eastern cooking.

O   8. This ingredient is used in place of butter or lard for cooking.

S   9. These are used to give a delicate flavor to foods.

K   10. Foods given this description are considered lawful to eat according to the Islamic religion.

E   11. This dish contains a mixture of ground meat and seasonings wrapped in grape leaves or stuffed into vegetables.

A   12. Middle Eastern people serve this at every meal.

B   13. This is a grain product made from whole wheat that has been cooked, dried, partly debranned, and cracked.

C   14. With the exception of Iran, this beverage is served throughout the Middle East.

T   15. This is the main beverage of Iran.

Middle East Regional Cuisine

Name ____

Date ____________________________ Period ____________

Answer the following questions about similarities and distinctions among the regional cuisines of the Middle East.

1. What food is forbidden by religions widely practiced in all Middle Eastern countries? ______________
   Pork is forbidden by religions widely practiced in all Middle Eastern countries.

2. What is the staple meat in the Middle East? Lamb is the staple meat in the Middle East.

3. What dairy product is served throughout the Middle East in a variety of dishes? ______________
   Yogurt is a dairy product served throughout the Middle East in a variety of dishes.

4. What are the staple grains in the Middle East? Wheat and rice are the staple grains in the Middle East.

5. What are the staple legumes in the Middle East? Beans, lentils, and chickpeas are the staple legumes in the Middle East.

6. Identify each of the countries indicated on the map.

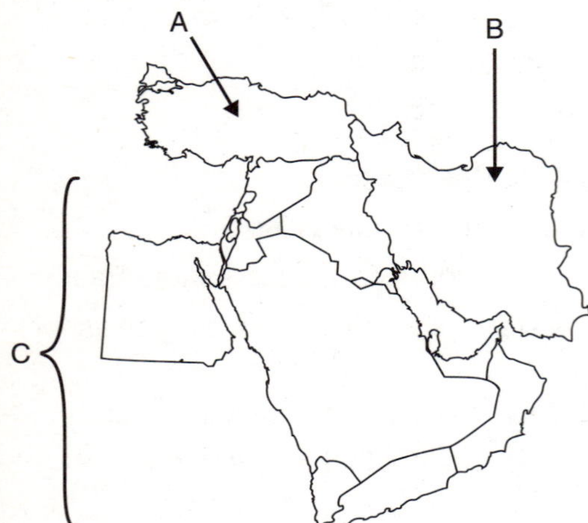

A. Turkey

B. Iran

C. (Group of countries) Arab states

Match the countries in the map with each of the following foods. Place the letter of the country that is most closely associated with each food in the blank to the left of the number.

A	7. halva		A	16. döner kebab
C	8. shrak		B	17. khoresh
C	9. torshi		C	18. mazza
B	10. tea		A	19. khave
C	11. kibbi		C	20. hummus
B	12. chelo		C	21. tabbouleh
A	13. cacik		A	22. kurabiye
C	14. arak		B	23. caviar
A	15. rahat lokum		B	24. polo

Israeli Culture and Cuisine

Activity C   Name ____

Chapter 32   Date _______________________   Period ____________

Read the following statements about the culture and cuisine of Israel. Circle *T* if the statement is true. Circle *F* if the statement is false.

(T) F   1. Jerusalem is called the *Holy City* by Christians, Jews, and Muslims.

(T) F   2. Lack of rainfall during the summer months makes irrigation necessary for the production of most crops in Israel.

T (F)   3. Members of a kibbutz receive wages for their work.

T (F)   4. Israel imports most of the fruits and vegetables consumed there.

(T) F   5. The land on which Israel is established used to be called Palestine.

T (F)   6. Jewish holidays always begin and end at dawn.

(T) F   7. The seder is a traditional meal of symbolic foods served on the first evening of Passover.

(T) F   8. Jewish cuisine is multinational.

T (F)   9. Foods that are not prepared according to Jewish dietary laws are considered to be kosher.

(T) F   10. According to Jewish dietary laws, foods such as shellfish, swine, and wild fowl cannot be consumed.

(T) F   11. According to Jewish dietary laws, all animals and fowl must be slaughtered by a licensed slaughterer known as a shohet.

T (F)   12. Milchig and fleishig foods are frequently cooked together to carefully blend the flavors.

T (F)   13. Pareve foods include dairy foods and meats.

T (F)   14. Gefilte is a popular chicken dish.

(T) F   15. Homemade noodles and dumplings are frequent additions to soups, main dishes, and puddings.

(T) F   16. Kugels may be served as side dishes or desserts, depending on the ingredients.

T (F)   17. Tzimmes are combinations of meats, vegetables, and fruits that are quickly fried for a fresh, light flavor.

T (F)   18. Blintzes are layered, torte-like cakes filled with whipped cream.

T (F)   19. Knishes are a type of fish.

(T) F   20. Matzo meal, made from unleavened bread, is used to make knaidlach, mandlen, and latkes.

(T) F   21. Challah is a rich, egg bread that is usually braided and served at Jewish holiday meals.

(T) F   22. Felafel, a mixture of ground chickpeas, bulgur, and spices that is formed into balls and deep-fried, has become one of Israel's national dishes.

(T) F   23. An Israeli delicacy known as leben is a type of cheese made from sour milk.

T (F)   24. Couscous is an Israeli dish with Russian origins.

(T) F   25. Sabra, an Israeli liqueur that has the flavor of the Jaffa orange, is often used to make rich desserts.

An African Food Guide

Activity D Name ___________________________

Chapter 32 Date _________________________ Period ____________

Following is a list of some African foods and ingredients. Indicate the food group to which each item belongs by writing the associated letter in the appropriate section of the platter below. Then answer the questions at the bottom of the page.

A. cassava
B. chicken
C. dates
D. figs
E. goat

F. ground nuts
G. guava
H. injera
I. kesra
J. lamb

K. okra
L. palm oil
M. papaya
N. pita bread
O. plantains

P. rice
Q. seafood
R. sugarcane
S. tomatoes
T. yams

1. Which MyPlate food group is not well represented by this list? _dairy_

2. How would following a traditional African meal pattern affect a person's efforts to get recommended daily intakes from the MyPlate food groups? ______________________________

   A traditional African meal pattern includes just two meals a day. This means a person would need to consume larger portions from each food group at each meal.

3. Why do you think snacking is popular in Africa? ______________________________

   Snacks would help relieve hunger and provide nutrients between the two daily meals.

4. Write a menu for an African meal that includes foods from the food guide above.

   (Answers will vary.)

Asia

Russian Culture and Cuisine

Activity A Name ____

Chapter 33 Date ___________________________ Period ____________

Complete the following statements about Russian culture and cuisine by using the words that follow to fill in the blanks in the numbered items below.

beef stroganov	schi	kulich	kisel
borscht	zakuska	pirozhki	ouba
czar	blini	shashlik	samovar
koumys	caviar	queen cake	smetana
paskha	kasha	chicken Kiev	

1. Pancakes made from buckwheat flour, which are called __blini__, are sold in parks during the Festival of Winter.

2. A Russian dessert with Slavic origins is __queen cake__, which is apples and cherries baked between layers of sweet pastry and topped with meringue.

3. A special piece of equipment used to make Russian tea is the __samovar__.

4. In 1547, Ivan the Terrible became the first __czar__, or ruler, of Russia.

5. A staple food of Russian peasants was __kasha__, which was made from raw grain that was fried and then simmered until tender.

6. Russian appetizers are called __zakuska__.

7. A food made from processed, salted eggs of large fish is called __caviar__.

8. Cabbage soup called __schi__ is one of the most popular Russian soups.

9. Russians often top __borscht__, their well-known beet soup, with a dollop of sour cream.

10. A clear fish broth called __ouba__ is popular in Russia.

11. Cubes of marinated lamb grilled on skewers is a regional dish called __shashlik__.

12. Tender strips of beef, mushrooms, and a seasoned sour cream sauce are used to make __beef stroganov__.

13. Pounded chicken breasts are wrapped around pieces of butter and then deep fried until golden brown to make __chicken Kiev__.

14. __Pirozhki__ are pastries filled with protein-based or sweet fillings.

15. Sour mare's milk, or __koumys__, is one of several dairy products that are important in Russian cooking.

16. Pureed fruit, called __kisel__, was a dessert eaten by Russian peasants.

17. A rich cheesecake molded into a pyramid and decorated with the letters XB is the Russian Easter dessert called __paskha__.

18. __Kulich__ is a tall, cylindrical yeast bread filled with fruits and nuts that is served as part of the Easter celebration of the Russian Orthodox Church.

Indian Culture and Cuisine

Activity B **Name** _______________________________

Chapter 33 **Date** _____________________ **Period** ___________

Read the following statements about the culture and cuisine of India. Circle *T* if the statement is true. Circle *F* if the statement is false.

(T) F 1. India is the seventh largest country in the world.

T (F) 2. In India, the soil in the Ganges River basin is poor and produces only one small crop yield each year.

(T) F 3. Foreign invasions lasting many centuries contributed to the variety of racial strains and more than 700 languages and dialects in India today.

(T) F 4. The social system known as the caste system developed from Hinduism.

T (F) 5. An Indian thanksgiving celebration for the winter harvest of rice is called the Janmashtami Festival.

(T) F 6. Hindu people celebrate the Ganesha Festival by offering candy and fruit to statues of an elephant-headed god.

(T) F 7. Rice is the major crop grown in India.

T (F) 8. Cattle are raised in India primarily for meat.

T (F) 9. India's cuisine is not influenced by climate and geography.

T (F) 10. The foods of Northern India are hotter than the foods of Southern India.

(T) F 11. In Northern India where wheat grows, bread sometimes takes the place of rice at meals.

(T) F 12. Religion has been a major influence on the development of Indian cuisine.

(T) F 13. Hindus do not eat beef because the cow is considered sacred.

(T) F 14. Most Hindus are vegetarians.

(T) F 15. Muslims cannot eat pork.

T (F) 16. Curry is a sweet made from semolina.

(T) F 17. India's coastline provides a variety of fish, which are dried, marinated, and smoked.

(T) F 18. Many Indian meat dishes are made with mutton.

(T) F 19. Many Indian dishes are cooked in ghee (clarified butter).

T (F) 20. Indian cooks use only a few spices in cooking.

T (F) 21. Chutneys are mixtures of spices used to make curries.

(T) F 22. Indians make many of their sweets from milk.

(T) F 23. A tandoor is a clay oven often used in Northern India.

(T) F 24. Korma is a cooking technique in which foods are braised, usually in yogurt.

(T) F 25. Vinegar and spices create the hot, slightly sour flavor in foods prepared using the vindaloo technique of cooking.

(T) F 26. Chasnidarth is an Indian version of the Chinese sweet and sour.

T (F) 27. At Indian meals, dishes are served one at a time in special courses.

(T) F 28. At Indian meals, diners help themselves to the food by using their fingers.

China Match

Name ______________________________________

Date ______________________________ Period ____________

Match the descriptions on the left related to the culture and cuisine of China with the terms they describe on the right. Place the correct letters in the corresponding blanks to the left of each number.

H	1.	Historically, most of China's people have crowded within this geographic region.
M	2.	When the Chinese Communists gained control in 1949, they gave the country this name.
Q	3.	This is the most widely celebrated festival in China.
G	4.	This midsummer occasion is celebrated by holding boat races and eating rice cakes that have been wrapped in bamboo leaves.
O	5.	This is China's chief agricultural product.
P	6.	The liberal use of this ingredient causes the typical Chinese diet to be high in sodium.
J	7.	This is an important seasoning in Chinese cooking.
B	8.	This common Chinese ingredient is a gelatinous, cream-colored cake made from soybeans.
U	9.	This versatile Chinese cooking utensil looks like a metal bowl.
R	10.	This piece of Chinese cooking equipment looks like a round, shallow basket with openings.
S	11.	This is the most common Chinese cooking method.
L	12.	This well-known Chinese roasted dish is rolled inside thin pancakes with scallions and hoisin sauce.
K	13.	This type of noodle is made from flour and eggs and resembles spaghetti.
T	14.	This mixture of deep-fried pork cubes, pineapple, and vegetables is served in a sweet-sour sauce.
I	15.	This is the Chinese version of an omelet.
A	16.	This popular Chinese dessert consists of cubes of almond-flavored gelatin garnished with fruit.
N	17.	The Chinese use this term for black tea because black is an unlucky color.
D	18.	This thick porridge made from rice or barley is often served for breakfast in China.
F	19.	The Chinese enjoy these steamed dumplings filled with meat, fish, vegetables, or sweet fruit as a snack.
C	20.	The Chinese use these eating utensils for all dishes except soup and finger foods.

A. almond float
B. bean curd
C. chopsticks
D. congee
E. curved spatulas
F. dim sum
G. Dragon Boat Festival
H. Eastern China
I. egg foo yung
J. ginger root
K. lo mein
L. Peking duck
M. People's Republic of China
N. red tea
O. rice
P. soy sauce
Q. Spring Festival
R. steamer
S. stir-frying
T. sweet and sour pork
U. wok

Focus on Japan

Name _______________________

Date _______________________   Period ___________

Imagine one of the associates from your Japan office has a beautiful video about her homeland. You want to show it to your coworkers so they will be more knowledgeable about life in Japan when dealing with Japanese clients. However, the video is narrated in Japanese. Use information in the text to help write a narration for the video scenes described in the following. Be sure to use descriptive language that will really bring the visual images to life. Write your responses in the space provided.

1. An aerial shot of the Japanese islands sweeps down to show the mountains and then passes over a highly populated urban area.

    (Answers will vary.)

2. A shot of a sunny terraced hillside dissolves into a shot of the same hillside being pounded by heavy rains and strong winds.

    (Answers will vary.)

3. A close-up shot shows cherry blossoms growing on a tree. As the camera angle widens, the shot pans down to show a family picnicking under the blooming tree.

    (Answers will vary.)

4. A medium-long shot shows Japanese farmers working in a rice paddy.

    (Answers will vary.)

5. A pan shot through a farmers' market shows vendors selling a wide variety of fresh fruits and vegetables.

    (Answers will vary.)

6. A long shot shows a fisherman on a boat tossing his day's catch onto the dock.

    (Answers will vary.)

(Continued)

7. A pan shot down a busy street moves through the door of a restaurant and back into the restaurant kitchen. Then a medium shot shows a chef quickly and skillfully carving vegetables into the shapes of animals and arranging them on a buffet tray.

   (Answers will vary.)

8. Another medium shot in the restaurant sequence shows a second chef cleaning and preparing blowfish.

   (Answers will vary.)

9. A third shot in the sequence shows another chef wrapping strips of seaweed around balls of cooked rice filled with vegetables.

   (Answers will vary.)

10. A new sequence begins in a family's home with a medium-long shot of family members gathering around a low table. Then a close-up shot shows the mother preparing food on a small grill built into the center of the table.

    (Answers will vary.)

11. The dinner sequence continues with a medium shot of the father removing the cover from his rice bowl. This is followed by a medium shot of a child eating with chopsticks.

    (Answers will vary.)

12. The final scene of the dinner sequence is a medium shot of the mother pouring tea.

    (Answers will vary.)

Chinese and Japanese Cuisine

Activity E   **Name** ____

Chapter 33   **Date** _____________________   **Period** ____________

The following statements relate to basic ingredients, cooking methods, utensils, serving customs, and meal patterns that are part of Chinese and Japanese cuisine. If a statement relates to Chinese cuisine, write *C* in the blank to the left of the number. If a statement relates to Japanese cuisine, write *J* in the blank. If a statement relates to both Chinese and Japanese cuisines, write *B* in the blank. Then answer the questions that follow.

  B   1. Sweet desserts are reserved for special occasions.

  J   2. Aesthetic appearance is an important element of the cuisine.

  C   3. A cleaver is used to perform all cutting tasks when preparing food.

  B   4. Fish is more important to the diet than meat.

  B   5. Three meals are typically served each day.

  C   6. Soup is eaten with spoons.

  J   7. A traditional ceremony is performed when tea is served.

  J   8. Diners show appreciation for the cook's skill by smacking their lips or making sucking sounds.

  C   9. Five-spice powder is an important seasoning.

  B   10. Foods are eaten with chopsticks.

  B   11. Steaming is one of the main cooking methods.

  J   12. A small, soft towel called an oshibori is used instead of a napkin.

  C   13. The wok is used as a versatile cooking utensil.

  J   14. Foods are cooked on a hibachi.

  B   15. Tea is the national drink.

  B   16. Rice is a basic ingredient.

  J   17. Broiling is a common cooking method.

  C   18. Stir-frying is the most common cooking method.

19. What similarities exist between the cuisines of China and Japan?

    (Answers will vary.)

20. What characteristics make Chinese cuisine distinct?

    (Answers will vary.)

21. What characteristics make Japanese cuisine distinct?

    (Answers will vary.)